Beans!

Peas and Lentils

Beans!

Peas and Lentils

h.f.ullmann

Contents

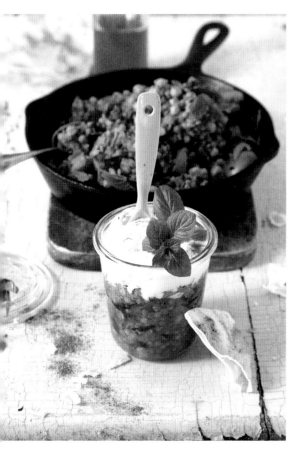
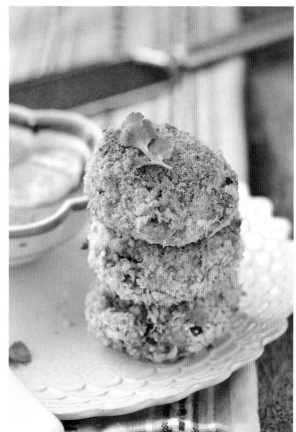
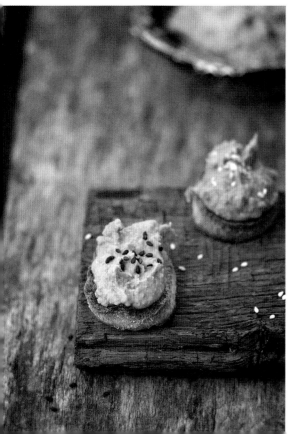
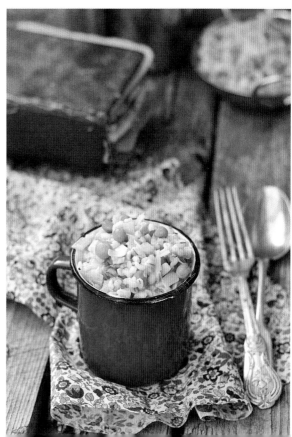

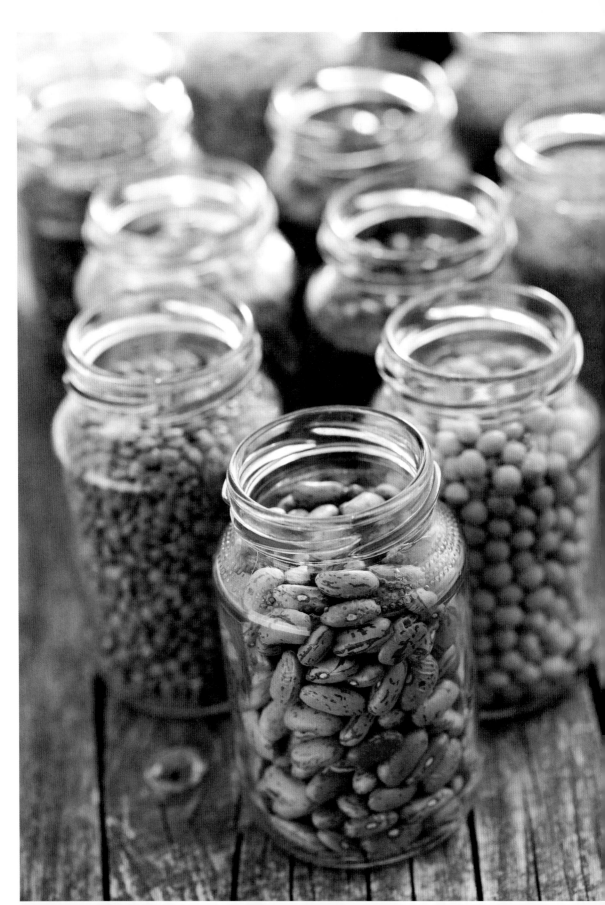

Pulses–popular as ever

Pulses, also known as legumes, include chickpeas, lentils, beans, peas, soybeans, and even peanuts, are known to have been cultivated worldwide for thousands of years. In Europe, they have long been a classic ingredient in traditional dishes, especially hearty stews. Consequently, as popular tastes began increasingly to veer away from filling dishes of this kind, pulses began to feature less and less as part of our daily diet. However, the past few years have–quite rightly–seen pulses experience something of a comeback. No longer confined to heavy stews, they are now an increasingly popular ingredient in salads, spreads, delicious curries, and even soups. Thanks to the huge range of dried beans, peas, lentils, and chickpeas available on today's supermarket shelves, pulses are now readily available and offer plenty of variety. As an alternative to dried pulses, which need a lot of soaking and lengthy cooking before use (see p. 12), they are also available canned and ready-cooked, or, in the case of green beans and peas, fresh or frozen. The choice is considerable and includes something to suit everyone's taste.

Surpassed only by daisies and orchids, legumes constitute the third largest family of flowering plants worldwide, numbering around 700 genera and 18,000 species. They are also one of the most important cultivated plants with approximately 150 million tons being grown each year throughout the world. No one knows for sure precisely where they originated, but Asia, the Near East, and Latin America are thought to be the most probable sources. It is likely that several species developed more or less simultaneously in different regions. Archeological finds show that peas, for example, were already being cultivated in Europe as long ago as 4,500 BC. Chickpeas, the name of which is derived from the Latin "cicer" (pea), are believed to have been cultivated in the Near East and Southeast Asia as far back as 10,000 BC and to have spread from there to Mexico. Nor must we forget the Ancient Egyptians in this respect: they were already growing lentils about 7,000 years ago. Nowadays, most cultivation areas are found in Africa, Asia, North, and South, America. From here, they are exported all over the world and are an important element in the world's food supply especially in poorer regions of the world.

Miniature power packs

Pulses are cultivated primarily for their edible seeds. As is the case with all plants, the seed is a veritable powerhouse of energy, containing in concentrated form all the important nutrients necessary to create a new plant. If we consider the substances and compounds contained in peas and lentils, etc., it is perfectly obvious that these foods represent veritable power packs which can considerably benefit our bodies.

To begin with, they contain a large amount of valuable vegetable protein. This makes them a particularly important element in a vegetarian diet. Supplemented with grain or milk, they provide more or less the same amount of protein as chicken, for example. In addition, they also supply satiating carbohydrates as well as up to 20 percent of dietary fiber yet are low in calories and nitrate. As far as providing protein is concerned, lentils are the front runners: not only do they supply the most protein but also the lowest amounts of carbohydrates. Meanwhile, in the fiber stakes, beans beat all other types of vegetable.

Since pulses take longer to digest, due to their high fiber content, the feeling of fullness they produce lasts longer. Furthermore, this digestive process also boosts stomach, gall bladder, and liver activity, which in turn speeds up the metabolism and supplies energy. Pulses are consequently not only a popular component of dieting programs but are equally good for general intestinal health. Another positive effect of slower digestion is that eating pulses does not cause a rapid increase or subsequent drop in blood sugar levels. Not only is this good for diabetics but regular consumption of pulses also reduces the risk of Type 2 diabetes. However, these are not the only effects that low-fat chickpeas, beans, and other pulses can have on our bodies.

Numerous studies have shown that even small portions of pulses each week can reduce cholesterol and high blood pressure as well as reduce the risk of heart disease, circulatory problems, and strokes. One study showed, for example, that a daily portion of 5 ounces/150 grams of cooked chickpeas could, within one month, noticeably reduce LDL cholesterol levels and consequently the cholesterol and triglyceride levels overall. However, it must be remembered that everyone's body will process and react to substances differently (see below), and other associated factors and medical conditions must always be taken into account. For most people, however, pulses are perfectly easy to digest and offer plenty of positive benefits. They contain lots of antioxidants, for example, and consequently help not only to slow down the skin aging process but also reduce the risk of cancer. A Japanese study, carried out over a period of seven years and involving over 43,000 people who carried an increased risk of cancer and whose diet was low in fiber, indicated that increasing the amount of dietary fiber led to a reduction in the risk of bowel cancer. The fiber supplied by pulses is also thought to reduce or even prevent the uptake of carcinogens, in other words, cancer-causing substances. Not only do the antioxidants contained therein combat the free radicals, which are major factors in causing cancer, but they can also slow down the development of arteriosclerosis. The darker the bean, the higher its content of anthocyanin, a substance also contained in fruits such as blueberries and blackcurrants. These powerful little pulses also contain nutrients such as iron, potassium, magnesium, phosphorus, and folic acid as well as vitamins A, C, E, and the B-vitamins B1, B2, and B6. Vitamin B1, in particular, is good for the nerves and makes us less susceptible to stress.

... but sadly, not right for everyone

No matter how wonderful the positive qualities of beans may sound, sayings such as "beans make their own kind of music" have not been coined for nothing. Beans do not necessarily agree with everyone as the gases produced during the breakdown of various substances have to find an escape route. One way of avoiding intestinal gas is only to use pulses which have been peeled as these contain less fiber. Dried varieties are also better in this respect. The indigestible substances are released from the pulses during soaking and subsequently discarded with the water in which they were soaked. Spices, such as aniseed, caraway seed, cumin, or fennel, can likewise aid digestion. Just keep trying out different types and preparation methods until you find what works for you.

Unfortunately, pulses also contain so-called purines which the body transforms into uric acid. Anyone suffering from gout or kidney disease should therefore consult a doctor as to whether it is advisable to eat pulses and, if so, in what quantity.

Kitchen basics

Fresh, frozen, canned, or dried—pulses are available in many different forms. They all have their own advantages and disadvantages and whichever type you choose will determine how much time you will need to spend in the kitchen.

Green beans, in particular, as well as wax beans, princess beans, French beans, and string beans, are readily available fresh. However, since they quickly lose this freshness, they should not be stored any longer than two days in the vegetable compartment of your refrigerator. Nor should they be stored next to apples, pears, or even tomatoes as these give off a gas which causes brown marks on the beans. You can extend the storage life of beans to some extent by blanching them briefly. Since beans contain phasin, they should not be eaten raw. Fresh beans should be crisp and unblemished by brown marks.

Before cooking, wash the beans well, top and tail the ends and, if necessary, remove any stringy fibers. If a plentiful harvest has left you with more beans than you can immediately use, the excess beans can be frozen—in which case, they should be cleaned as described above, blanched for approximately 3–5 minutes, then doused in cold water. Once they have been thoroughly drained, transfer them to a freezer bag or box and freeze. They can be stored in this way for 9 to 15 months. In the case of broad beans, snap open the pod and extract the individual beans. These can also be peeled, if so desired. Blanching for 5 minutes will make this task easier.

Fresh peas are likewise often available in supermarkets if you have not grown them in your own garden. Unlike beans, they can be eaten fresh and add that extra touch to salads. In the case of marrowfat peas, snap open the pod and extract the peas. Once they have been washed, they can either be eaten raw or blanched briefly. Since they only need a brief amount of cooking, they are usually not added to a dish until a few minutes before the end of cooking.

If using tender, sugar snap peas, cut off the base of the stalk and wash. They can be cooked from raw without any pre-boiling.

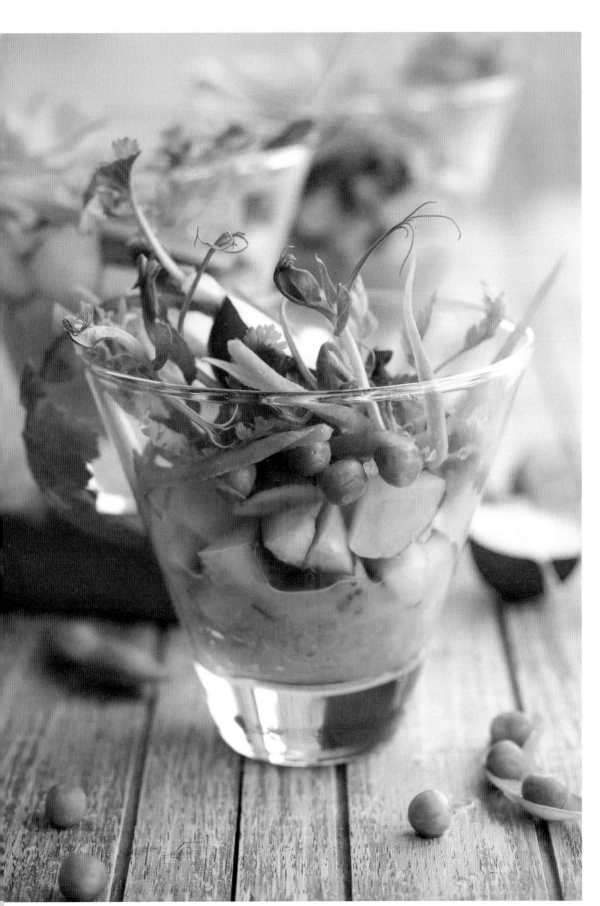

Beans and peas can also be found in the frozen food section of your local supermarket. Since they just need to be cleaned, blanched, and quickly frozen straight after harvesting, frozen peas, unlike canned vegetables, retain most of their nutrients. A further advantage is that you can keep a supply of frozen beans and peas in the freezer, from which smaller quantities can be extracted as and when they are needed. These will be ready to use with minimal preparation, requiring no defrosting beforehand and offering an excellent alternative to the fresh version.

Dried versus canned pulses

Dried lentils, like peeled, dried peas and a few smaller varieties of bean, do not need soaking before use. Nor do they need to cook for as long as some other varieties. There are a number of different varieties to choose from, depending on the dish in question: black Beluga lentils, brown mountain lentils, and green du Puy lentils tend to be smaller and remain firm during cooking. They are ideal for salads or as a side dish. Yellow and red lentils are peeled varieties and disintegrate into a mush when cooked. They are an integral part of Indian cuisine and need only approximately 15 minutes' cooking time. The larger varieties, such as lima/butter beans are floury and perfect for stews.

Dried chickpeas and most beans must be soaked before cooking. The length of soaking time is generally indicated on the packet and is usually around 12 hours. Before soaking, place the pulses in a bowl of water: any pulses which float to the surface should be removed as they may have been attacked by insects or deteriorated as a result of being stored for too long. The remaining pulses should then be rinsed well under running water to wash off any dust and they should also be checked for any residue of grit or small stones.

To soak, place the pulses in a bowl filled with water, basing the quantities on a ratio of one part pulses to about three parts of water. Once soaked overnight, pulses should be rinsed before cooking in fresh water.

To cook, place the rinsed pulses in a large saucepan and cover with fresh water. Bring to a boil, then reduce the heat, partly cover the pan with a lid, then simmer over a low heat until tender. Make sure the saucepan is large enough to cope with all the foam produced during cooking. Keep skimming off the foam as it collects, adding more hot water, if necessary. How long the beans take to cook will depend on their size and vary between 45 minutes and 2 hours.

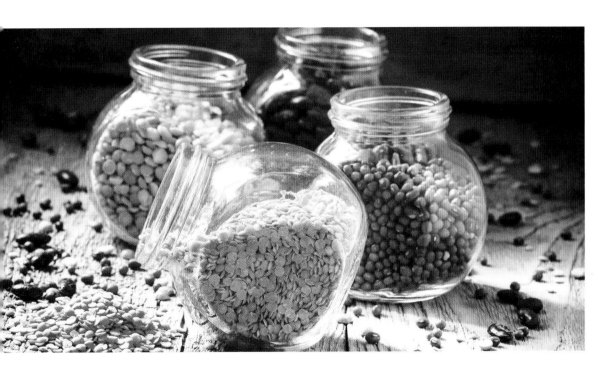

Chickpeas will likewise take about 2 hours to cook. Soaking the pulses for longer will reduce the cooking time. Using a pressure cooker can also save a great deal of time: even without soaking, beans and chickpeas will be cooked and tender within approximately 30–40 minutes. It is important not to add salt or acidic ingredients until just before the end of cooking time as they can prevent the pulses from cooking properly.

Dried pulses should be stored in a tightly sealed container and kept in a cool, dark, dry place. Stored in this way, they can keep for several years.

Canned pulses are a good alternative if you want to avoid lengthy soaking and cooking procedures or prefer not to have to plan things so far in advance. These are pre-cooked and can be used straight from the can. It is a matter of personal preference whether you discard the liquid or not. Anyone who suffers from flatulence is advised to drain the pulses and rinse them under running water. This will help to reduce the effects of intestinal gas.

When buying canned pulses, check that they do not contain any preservatives or additives. Make sure that the cans are not dented or damaged in any way. A dent may indicate that the inner coating of the can has been ruptured, causing the can to react with the contents and encourage the growth of mold, etc. If using jars of pulses, make sure that the lid is not damaged or dented otherwise the vacuum can no longer be guaranteed.

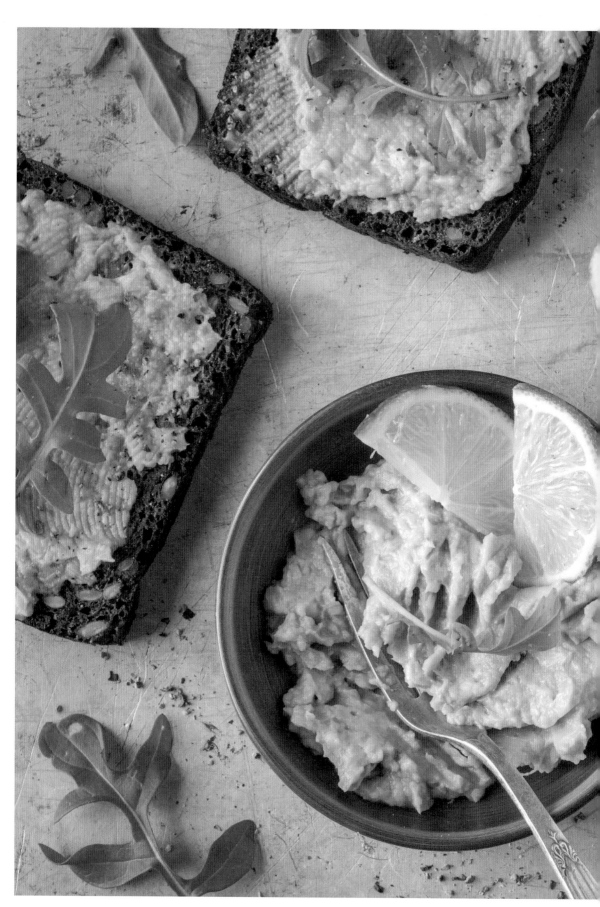

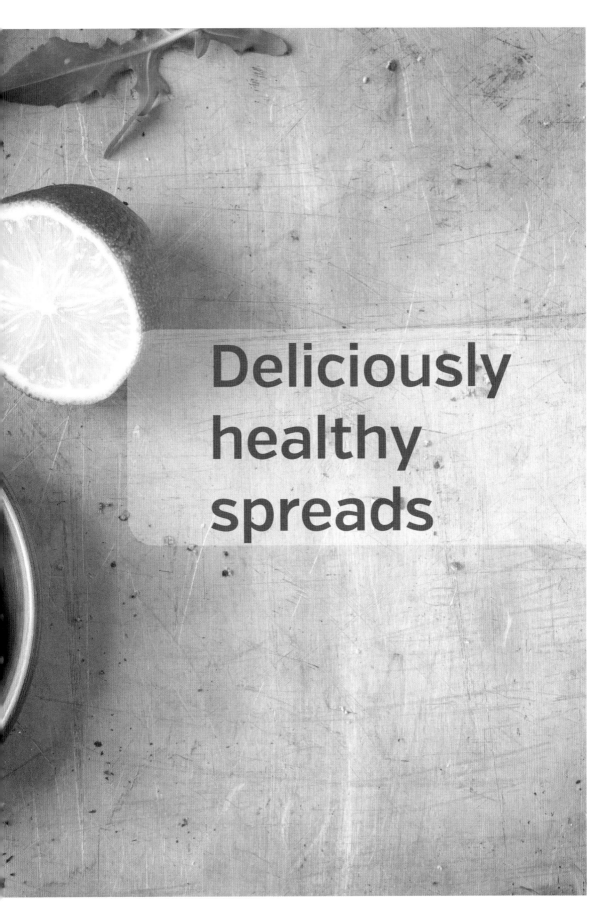

Deliciously healthy spreads

Beet and lentil spread

3 tbsp/35 g yellow
lentils
3½ tbsp/40 g red
lentils
⅔ cup/165 ml water
½ cup/50 g walnuts,
shelled
½ cup/100 g cooked
beets
1 tbsp sunflower oil
1 tbsp apple vinegar
½ tsp allspice
1 level tsp salt
freshly ground black
pepper

Place the lentils and water in a saucepan and bring
to a boil. Simmer for 20 minutes over a very low
heat. Turn off the heat and leave the lentils to soak
for a further 10–15 minutes until very soft.

Chop the walnuts, setting aside a few for the
garnish. Blend together with all the remaining
ingredients thoroughly in a food processor, then
place in the refrigerator to chill.

Tip
The above amount will probably be too much for
one person as the spread will only keep for a few
days. However, it is ideal for freezing. Provided
it does not contain any raw onion, freezing and
defrosting will have no detrimental effect on the
quality of the spread.

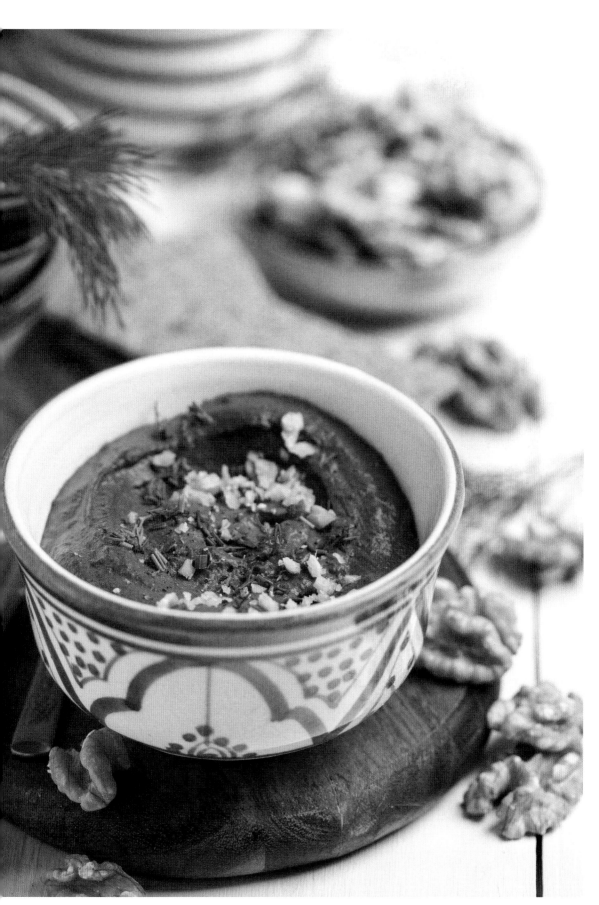

Fava bean and feta cream spread

3½ cups/750 g fava
bean pods (broad
beans)
2½ oz/75 g feta
1 tsp honey (wild
honey, if possible)
1 tsp lemon juice
12 fresh basil leaves,
depending on size
salt, to taste

Shell the fava beans (producing about 1½ cups/
225 g of shelled beans), then cook in a saucepan
with little water for around 10 minutes. Drain the
beans, leave to cool until just warm, then squeeze
gently to pop the beans out of their skins.

Place the beans in a tall, narrow blender bowl,
add the feta, cut into small pieces, add the honey
and lemon juice, then purée the ingredients into a
smooth paste.

Rinse the basil leaves, pat dry, and chop finely.
Add salt, to taste, then blend into the fava-and-
feta cream mixture.

Set the mixture aside to cool, transfer into jars,
and store in the refrigerator.

Tip
This fava-and-feta cream spread will keep in the
refrigerator for about three weeks. However, it
is best eaten as soon as possible as the basil
flavor quickly disappears. Alternatively, make the
spread without the basil initially, blending in freshly
chopped basil leaves just before each serving. The
spread can also be frozen without the basil.

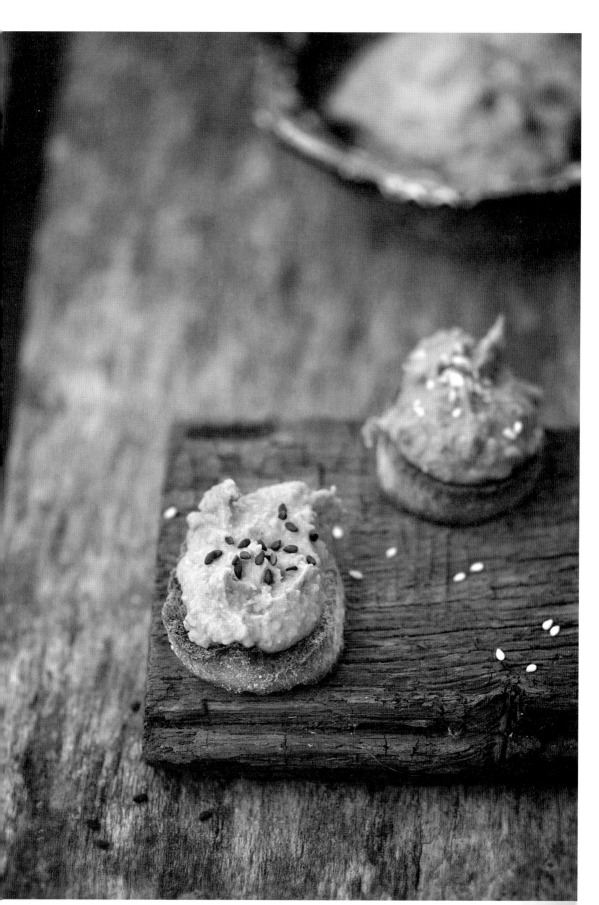

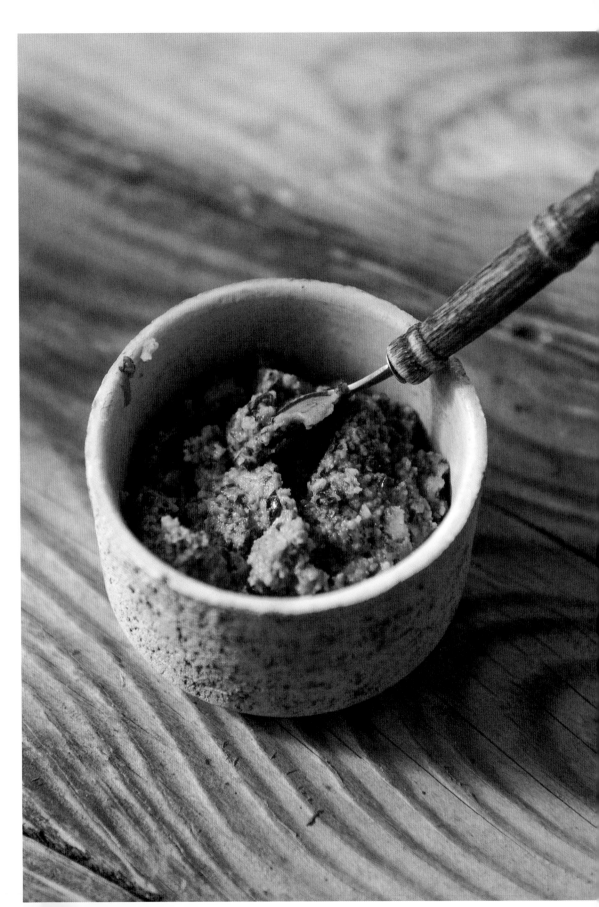

Eggplant and bean cream dip

1 tbsp olive oil
1 lb/500 g eggplants
1 can kidney beans
½ bunch cilantro
1 tsp tahini (sesame
seed paste)
½ tsp turmeric
½ tsp cumin
1 tbsp lemon juice
salt, pepper

Pre-heat the oven to 425 F° (220 °C), then brush the inside of an ovenproof dish with olive oil.

Cut the eggplants in half and lay them, cut side facing down, in the dish. Pierce the skins in several places, then bake in the oven for about 45 minutes until extremely soft.

Meanwhile, drain the kidney beans and rinse in cold water. Roughly chop the cilantro leaves and stalks.

Leave the eggplants to cool a little, then scoop out the flesh with a spoon. Blend the eggplant flesh, kidney beans, cilantro, and tahini to a smooth purée.

Season the eggplant and bean cream to taste with turmeric, cumin, lemon juice, salt, and pepper. Store in the refrigerator until required.

Fruity lentil and juniper spread

1 large bay leaf
1 red onion (about
2 oz/50 g)
2½ tbsp/40 ml melted
ghee (for the vegan
version use olive oil)
1 tbsp finely chopped
soup vegetables
½ cup/100 g mountain
lentils (or small brown
lentils)
8 juniper berries
2 heaped tsp plum
purée
salt and freshly milled
black pepper to taste

Using a sharp kitchen knife, carefully make a few incisions along the leaf veins of the bay leaf. Peel and dice the onion. Heat the ghee or olive oil in a saucepan, add the onion, bay leaf, and chopped soup vegetables, sweat until the onion is translucent.

Drain and rinse the lentils in a sieve. Add the lentils and juniper berries to the onion mixture in the saucepan, add enough water to cover the ingredients by about ⅓ inch/1 cm of water, then bring to a boil. Cook over a medium heat, adding a little hot water occasionally, if necessary, to prevent the lentils from sticking and burning.

As soon as the lentils begin to disintegrate (this can take up to an hour), remove the pan from the heat, discard the bay leaf, then purée the ingredients into a smooth paste using a hand-held stick blender. Return the saucepan to the stovetop and continue to simmer the puréed ingredients over a moderate heat, stirring constantly, until the mixture thickens into a spreadable paste. It is important to bear in mind that the purée will thicken and become even firmer once it has cooled.

Place the lentil paste in a bowl with the plum purée, blend well and season to taste with salt and pepper. Leave the spread to cool, transfer to glass jars, then store in the refrigerator.

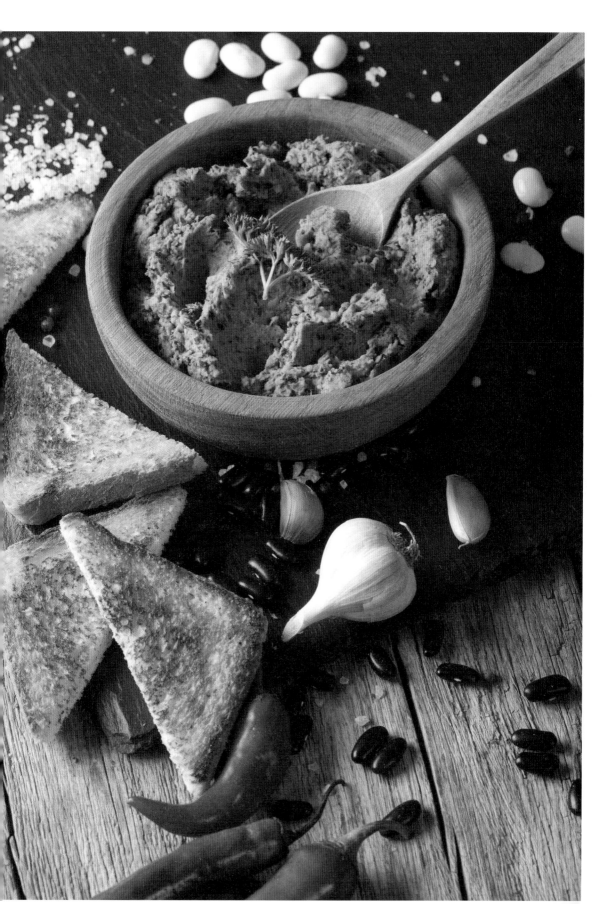

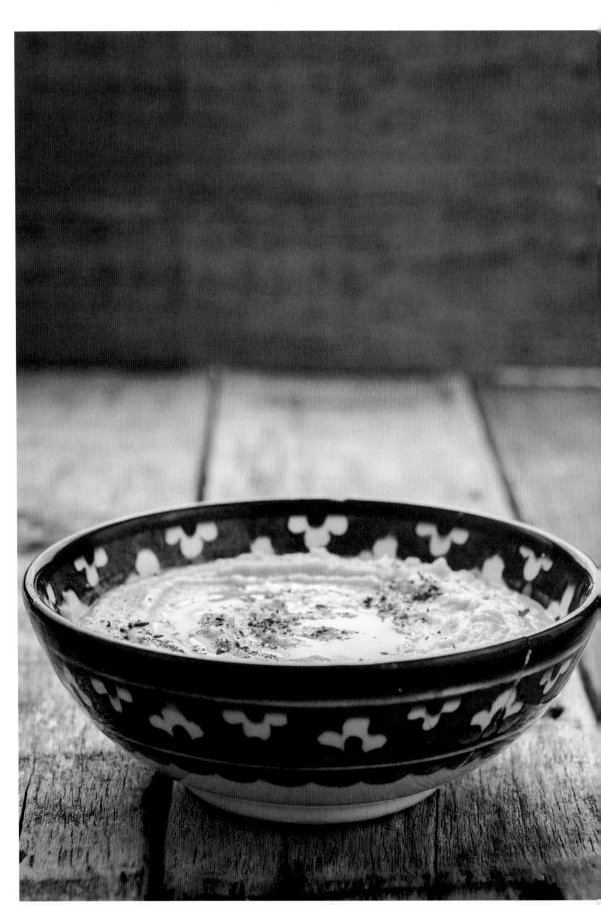

Fingerfood – hummus

Please note: Chickpeas must be soaked overnight. Canned chickpeas can be used straight from the can.

generous ½ cup + 1 tbsp/125 g dried chickpeas, or 1 whole can of chickpeas
1 garlic clove
2 tbsp tahini (sesame seed paste)
½ tsp cumin
1½ tbsp lemon juice
2 tbsp natural yogurt
salt, pepper, powdered paprika

Place the dried chickpeas in a bowl, cover with about ¾ in/2 cm of water and leave to soak overnight.

Next day, drain off the water, bring the chickpeas to a boil in 1 quart/1 liter of fresh water and simmer for about 15 minutes. (If using canned chickpeas, tip them into a sieve and rinse in fresh water.)

Peel the garlic clove, cut in half and remove the green core. Place the prepared chickpeas, tahini, garlic, and cumin in a food processor and blend into a creamy purée.

Finally, stir in the lemon juice and yogurt, then season to taste with salt, pepper, and paprika.

Hot and spicy chickpea and pumpkin spread

Please note: Dried chickpeas must be left to soak overnight.

¾ cup/150 g dried chickpeas
7 oz wedge/200 g Hokkaido pumpkin
2 garlic cloves
1 tsp chili oil
1 tsp harissa (hot seasoning paste)
salt

Cover the chickpeas with water and leave to soak overnight.

Next day, drain the chickpeas and bring to a boil in fresh water. Cover and cook over a low heat for about 60 minutes until soft. Drain and set aside to cool.

Pre-heat the oven to 325 °F (160 °C). Remove the seeds from the Hokkaido pumpkin, then slice or cut into large chunks. There is no need to remove the peel which is edible. In an ovenproof pan, bake the pumpkin pieces until tender, then set aside to cool. Peel and finely slice the garlic cloves. Warm the chili oil in a small skillet, stir in the garlic and sweat for at least 15 minutes.

Reserve a few chickpeas for decoration, then place the remaining chickpeas, pumpkin, and garlic oil mixture in a tall container and purée all the ingredients smoothly with a stick blender. Season to taste with salt and harissa, transfer to a serving bowl and garnish with the reserved chickpeas.

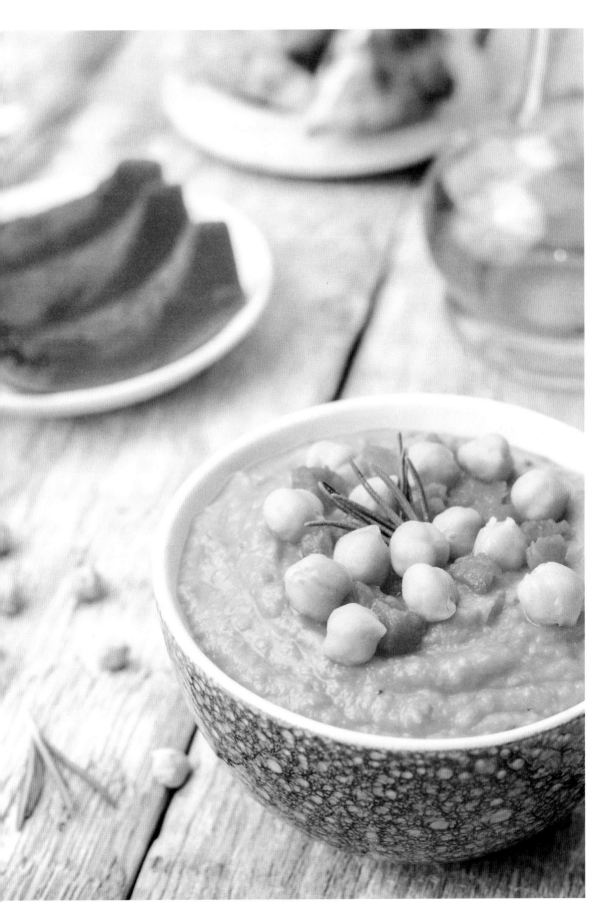

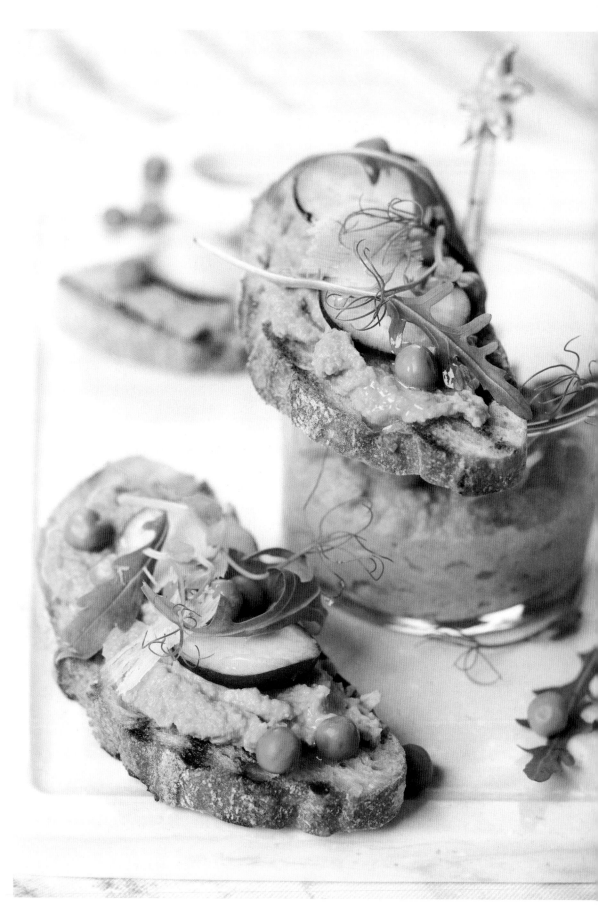

Pea and lime spread

Please note: The peas must be left to soak overnight.

1 cup/200 g dried, green peas
3½–4 oz/100 g leek
3½ tbsp/50 g butter (use 4 tbsp canola or sunflower oil for the vegan version)
1 level tsp wild garlic salt, or 3 stems fresh wild garlic (alternatively, 1 bunch chives)
2 tbsp lime juice
salt and freshly milled black pepper to taste

Tip
Transfer the spread to glass jars and store in the refrigerator.

Rinse the peas, place in a bowl and cover with about ¾ inch/2 cm of water. Leave to soak overnight.

Next day, drain the peas, remove the skins, and cut the peas in half. Wash and dry the leeks, cut in half lengthwise, and slice into thin semicircles. Heat a little of the butter or some of the oil in a large saucepan and gently fry the leeks.

Add the peas, and cover with about the same amount of water as before. Bring to a boil, cover, and cook over a low heat (this can take up to an hour). Skim off any foam which may appear in the early stages. Add a little hot water occasionally if necessary to prevent the peas sticking and burning. Once the peas begin to disintegrate, begin stirring and simmer until the resulting mixture develops the consistency of a spreadable paste.

Transfer the pea paste into a blender and purée until smooth. Cut the remaining butter into small pieces, add to the blender and allow to melt in the pea purée. (If using oil, wait until the purée has cooled down before adding to the mixture). Set the purée aside.

Finely slice the wild garlic or chives into thin rings. Stir the herbs and lime juice into the pea purée. Season to taste with pepper, and salt if required.

Indian lentil spread

generous ½ cup/100 g red lentils
1 large bay leaf
1 onion (about 2 oz/50 g)
1 garlic clove
¾ inch/2 cm fresh gingerroot
1 heaped tbsp coconut oil
1 lightly heaping tbsp finely diced soup vegetables
1 lightly heaping tsp mild curry powder
1 level tsp ground turmeric
salt, to taste

Rinse the red lentils in a sieve under cold, running water until it runs clear. Set aside.

Using a sharp kitchen knife, carefully make a few incisions along the veins of the bay leaf. Peel and dice the onion and garlic clove, then peel and finely grate the gingerroot.

Heat the coconut oil in a saucepan, add the onion, garlic, gingerroot, bay leaf, soup vegetables, curry powder, and turmeric and sweat all the ingredients over a moderate heat until the onion is translucent.

Add the lentils to the onion mixture, then cover with ¾ cup/200 ml of water. Cook over a medium heat until the lentils begin to disintegrate (about 25 minutes). Keep adding a little hot water occasionally, as necessary.

Discard the bay leaf and continue to simmer the lentil mixture over a medium heat, stirring constantly, until it develops a spreadable consistency. The paste will thicken and become firmer once it has cooled.

Transfer the lentil paste to a blender, purée until smooth, and season with salt to taste.

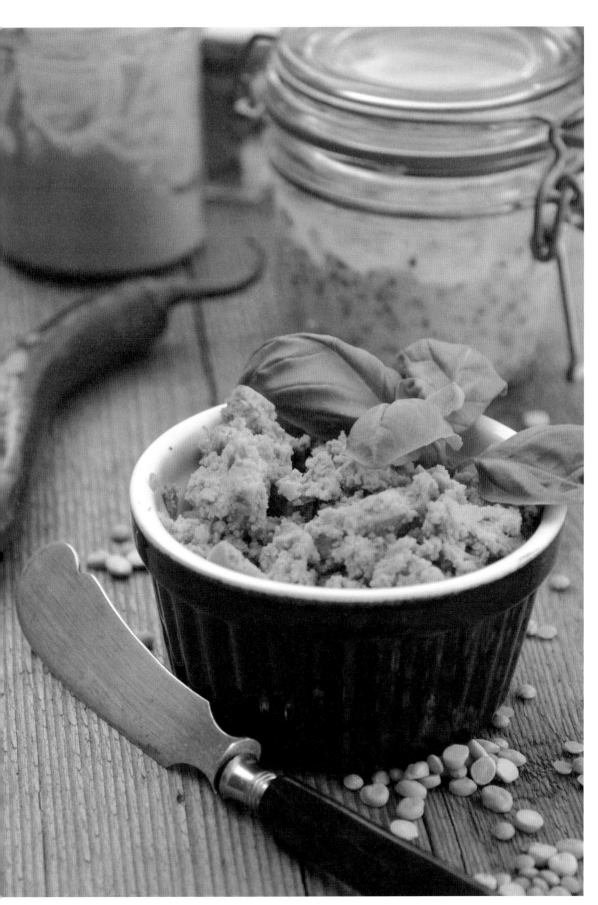

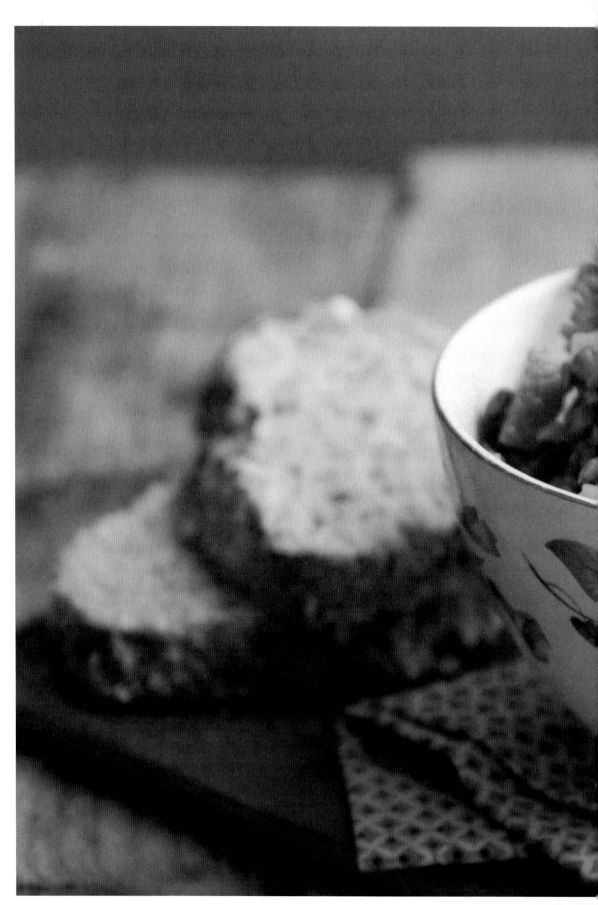

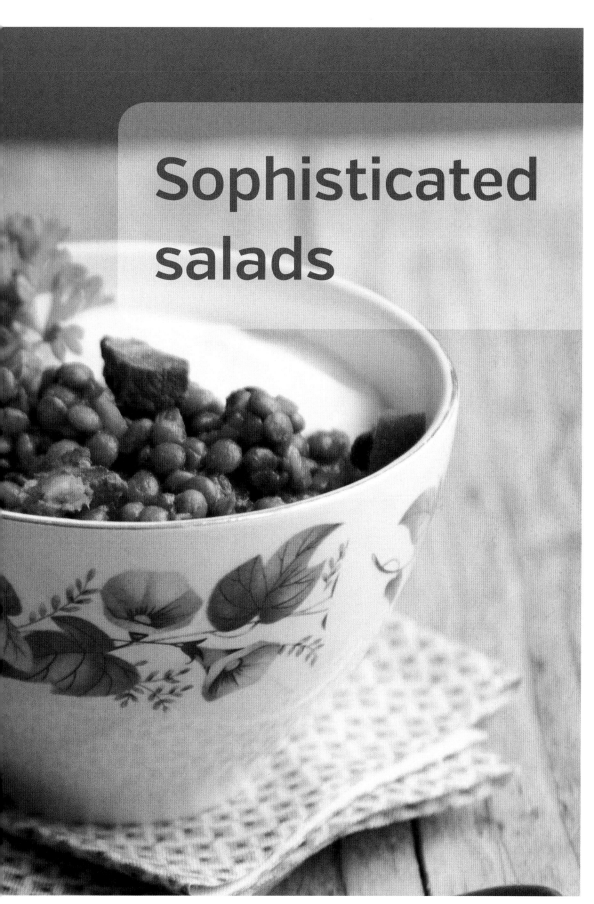

Sophisticated salads

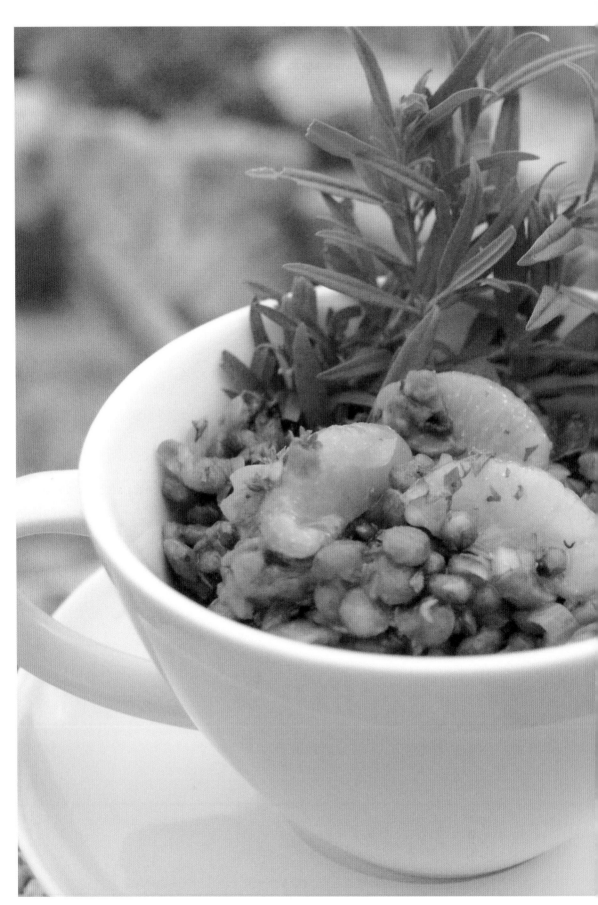

Hyssop and lentil salad

Serves 4

2 generous cups/500 g
lentils
2 quarts/2 liters water
1 bay leaf
3 sprigs thyme
1 red and 1 white onion
1½ cups/100 g button
mushrooms
1 handful each of
fresh hyssop, lovage,
parsley, chives
1 tbsp pickled green
peppercorns
salt, vinegar, oil
1 small can mandarin
oranges
edible flowers, for
decoration

Soak the lentils and cook according to packet instructions, with the bay leaf and thyme, but do not allow them to become too soft. Drain off the water, leave the lentils to cool, then discard the bay leaf and thyme.

Finely dice the onions and slice the mushrooms. Gently sauté both ingredients, in a little of the oil then leave to cool.

Finely chop the herbs. Mix all the above ingredients together, add the pickled peppercorns, vinegar, oil, and season to taste with salt.

Finish off by carefully stirring in the drained mandarin oranges. Serve the finished salad decorated with edible flowers.

Corn salad with beans and chickpeas

Serves 2

¼ cup/50 g dried chickpeas
generous ¼ cup/40 g dried kidney beans
1–2 packs/150 g corn salad, or mache
½ bunch radishes
2 tbsp flax seed oil
salt
freshly milled black pepper
2 tbsp sunflower seeds

Soak the chickpeas and kidney beans overnight in plenty of water. Tip into a sieve and drain, rinse well and place in a saucepan filled with fresh water. Bring to a boil, then cover and simmer over a low heat. Check whether the beans and chickpeas are tender, probably after 60 minutes, but check at intervals. If so, drain and set aside to cool.

Pick over the corn salad, then wash and spin dry. Clean, wash and thinly slice the radishes. Combine the corn salad, chickpeas, kidney beans, and radishes with the flax seed oil. Season with salt and pepper to taste, and garnish the salad with a sprinkling of sunflower seeds.

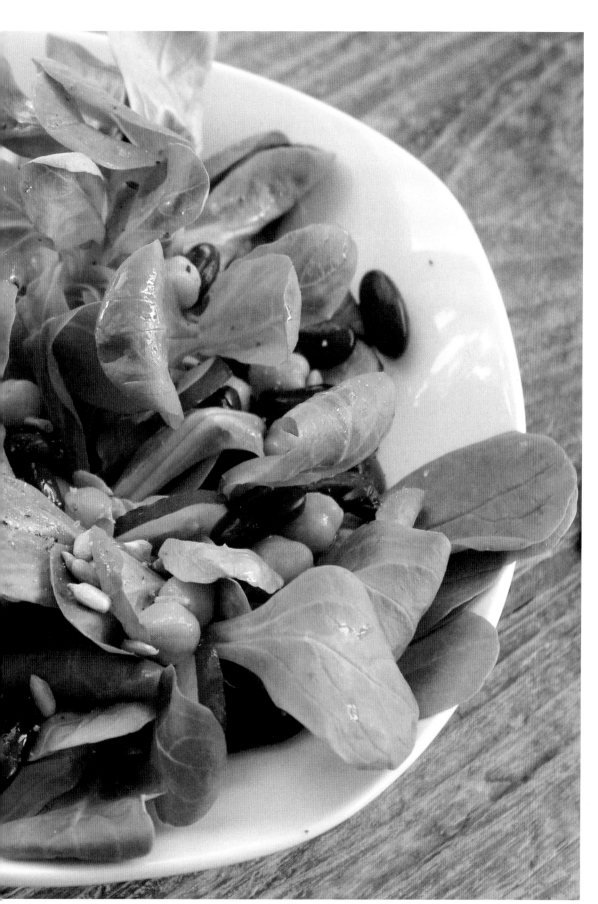

Aromatic bean salad

Serves 2

1 lb pack/400 g fresh
green beans
2 tsp coriander seeds
2 tsp black caraway
seeds
2 tbsp sesame seeds
1 red onion
2 garlic cloves
1 lemon
2–3 tbsp olive oil
salt
several fresh basil
leaves

Wash the beans under running water, drain, top and tail. Cook for about 10 minutes in boiling, salted water until firm to the bite. Plunge briefly in ice-cold water to retain their green color, then drain thoroughly.

Place the coriander and black caraway seeds with the sesame seeds in a dry, fat-free saucepan and toast over a low heat, stirring constantly. Remove the pan from the heat. Peel the onion, then slice into thin rings or dice finely. Peel and slice the garlic.

Using a sharp knife, peel the lemon rind and finely dice the flesh. Add the lemon flesh to the saucepan along with the onion, garlic, olive oil, beans, salt, to taste, and toasted seeds. Mix well without heating. Wash, dry, and finely chop the basil leaves and fold into the salad.

Tip
Add a few lovely, red radicchio leaves, cut into strips, mixing them into the bean salad to create a culinary treat which is both visually attractive and delicious to eat!

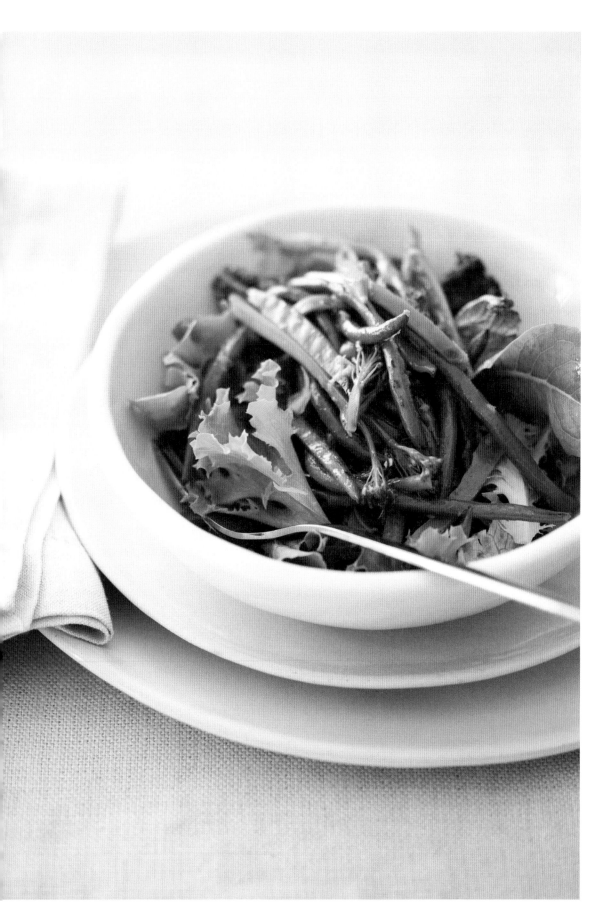

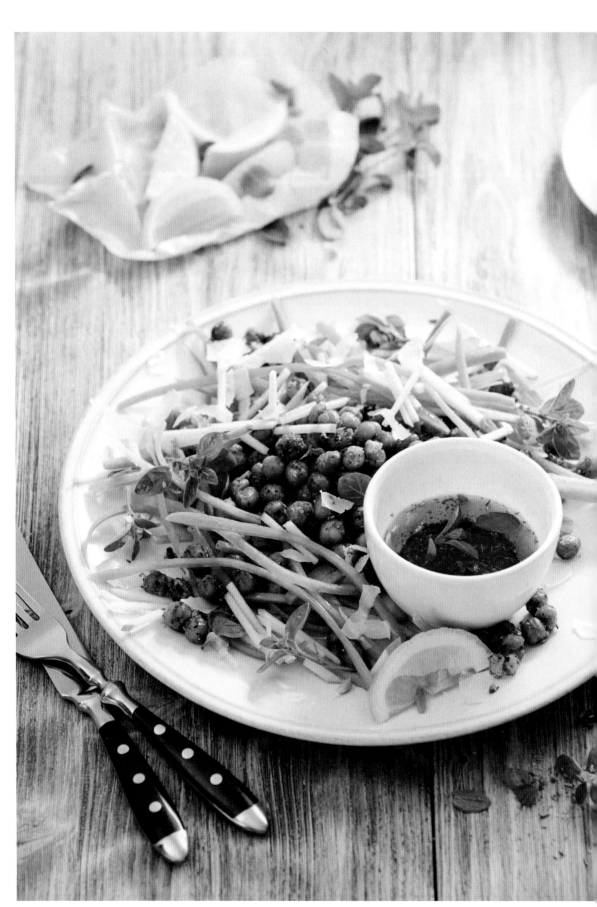

Moroccan chickpea salad

Serves 4

generous 1 lb/500 g
tender young carrots
3 tbsp olive oil
2 tsp ras el hanout
(Moroccan spice blend)
15 oz/400 g pre-
cooked chickpeas
½ bunch mint
1 lemon
1½ cups/200 g feta
salt, pepper

Pre-heat the oven to 400 °F (200 °C). Peel the carrots and slice diagonally into thin matchsticks. Sprinkle with 2 tablespoons of the olive oil and 1 teaspoon of the ras el hanout, then mix well. Spread the carrots over a baking sheet lined with parchment paper. Season with salt and pepper and mix well. Place in the pre-heated oven for 20–25 minutes.

Drain the chickpeas, rinse under cold, running water, then place in a salad bowl. Add the baked carrots to the chickpeas, drizzling the oil they were cooked in over the top.

Strip the mint leaves from their stems and finely chop. Squeeze the lemon, and stir the juice with the mint into the salad, together with the remaining ras el hanout and olive oil, if required. Season with salt and pepper to taste. Crumble the feta cheese and sprinkle over the salad before serving.

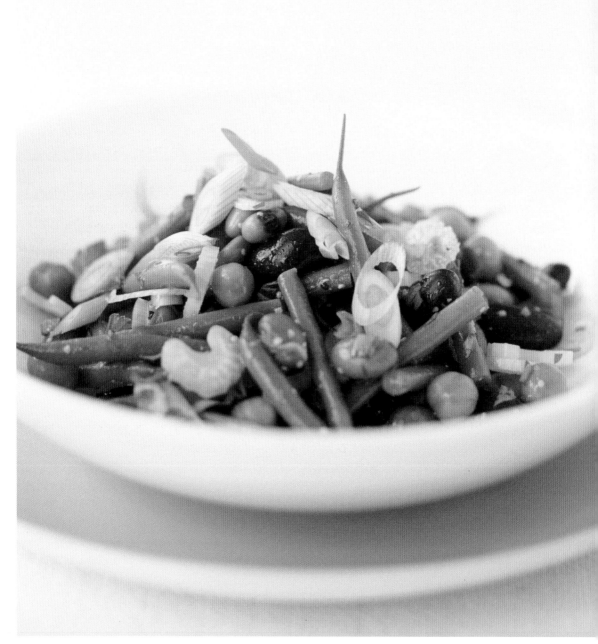

Mixed bean salad with summer vinaigrette

Serves 4

1 generous cup/200 g
borlotti or pinto beans
1 cup/200 g yellow wax
beans
1 cup/200 g green
beans
8 strips/100 g bacon
4 medium/100 g
shallots
oil for frying
1¼ cups/150 g fresh
redcurrants, or
chokeberries

For the vinaigrette
6 tbsp canola or
sunflower oil
3 tbsp white balsamic
vinegar
1 tsp Dijon mustard
1 bunch parsley
1 bunch savory
salt, freshly milled
black pepper

Soak the dried beans overnight. Drain and place in a clean saucepan, cover with fresh, cold water, bring to a boil, then cook for about one hour until tender but still firm to the bite (keep checking from time to time during cooking and add more hot water if necessary).

Blanch the green and yellow beans in salted water, then plunge briefly in ice-cold water.

Top and tail the wax beans and green beans, and remove any stringy fibers. Blanch in boiling, salted water for 5–10 minutes until just firm to the bite. Plunge in ice-cold water to retain the bright green color, then drain.

Dice the bacon and shallots into small pieces, fry in a little oil and sprinkle over the mixed beans.

Make a vinaigrette by blending the vinaigrette ingredients, then pour the dressing over the beans. Transfer the salad onto plates and garnish each portion with a spoonful of redcurrants or chokeberries, if available.

Mixed tomatoes with chickpeas

Serves 2

⅔ cup/140 g dried
chickpeas
about 24 individual/
400 g red and yellow
cherry tomatoes
½ lemon
4 tbsp olive oil
salt, freshly milled
black pepper
½ bunch basil
½ bunch parsley

Soak the chickpeas in water for 24 hours, then drain through a sieve and rinse. Place in a saucepan, cover with fresh water and cook for 30 to 40 minutes.

Meanwhile, wash and halve the cherry tomatoes. Squeeze the juice from the lemon. To make the dressing, combine the lemon juice, olive oil, salt and pepper, to taste. Wash the basil and parsley, pat dry, then strip the leaves off the stems and finely chop.

Once cooked, drain the chickpeas through a sieve, rinse in cold water and drain well. Tip into a salad bowl and mix with the cherry tomatoes. Stir in the dressing and serve sprinkled with the chopped basil and parsley.

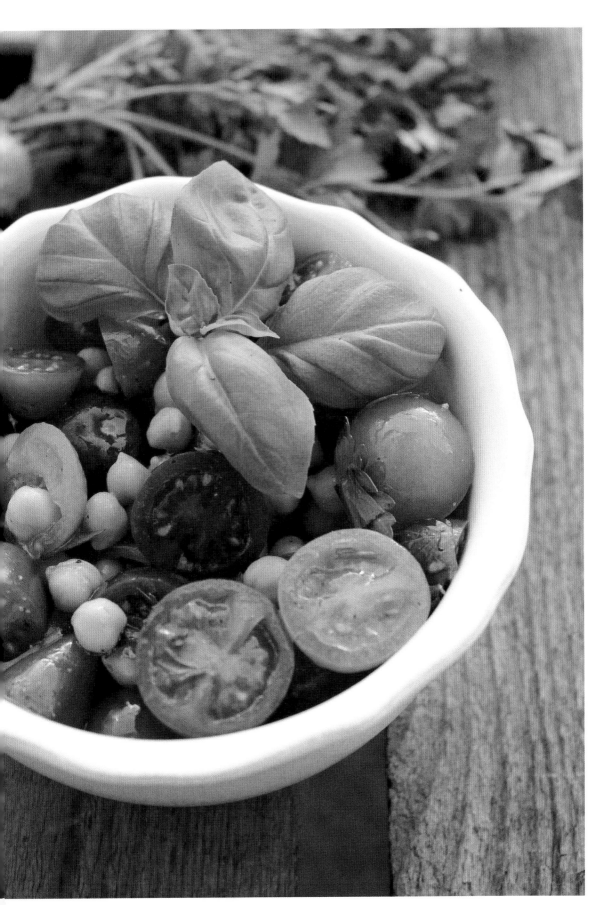

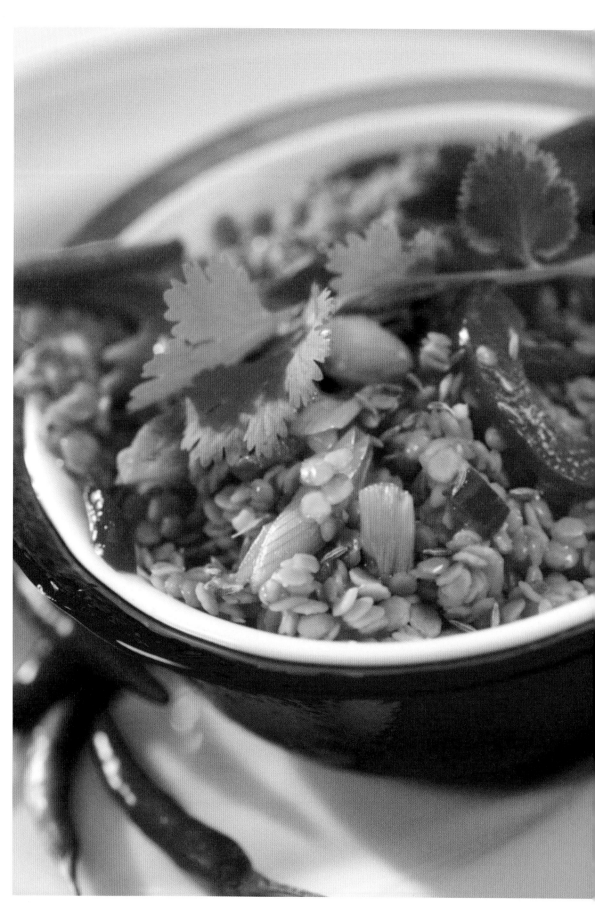

Red lentil salad with chile

Serves 4

1 cup/200 g red lentils
8–10 individual/125 g
cherry tomatoes
2 scallions
1 red bell pepper
½ cucumber
1¼ cups/250 g canned
pineapple chunks
1 small, red chile
pepper

For the dressing
4 tbsp balsamic
vinegar
1 tsp lemon juice
1 tbsp pineapple juice
5 tbsp olive oil
salt, freshly milled
black pepper
honey or mustard, to
taste

Cook the lentils for about 10 minutes over a low heat, then season with salt just before the end of cooking time. Tip into a sieve and drain thoroughly.

Cut the cocktail tomatoes into quarters, slice the scallions into thin rings. Dice the bell pepper. Remove the seeds from the cucumber (otherwise the salad will end up too watery), then cut into small cubes.

Drain the pineapple in a sieve, reserving some of the juice. Cut the chile pepper in half, remove the seeds, stalks, and white pith, then finely slice. Mix all the above ingredients together in a bowl. Mix the ingredients for the dressing.

Stir the dressing into the salad and mix all the ingredients together well. Leave to marinate for at least 30 minutes, then season to taste once more.

Beluga lentil salad

Serves 2

1 cup/240 ml vegetable
stock
generous ⅓ cup/80 g
dried Beluga lentils
1 red onion
2 tomatoes
1 avocado
juice of ½ lemon
2 tbsp flax seed oil
1–2 sprigs mint
few sprigs parsley
⅔ cup/50 g dried,
unsulfured apricots,
pitted
salt, freshly milled
black pepper

Bring the vegetable stock to a boil in a saucepan.
Place the Beluga lentils in a sieve and rinse in cold
water. Add them to the vegetable stock, cover and
cook for around 30 minutes, then drain.

Peel the onion, finely dice and put in a salad bowl.
Wash and finely dice the tomato flesh, discarding
the core, and add to the onion.

Peel the avocado and cut in half lengthwise. Use a
spoon to lift out the stone, finely dice the flesh and
add to the salad bowl. Sprinkle with lemon juice,
then drizzle the flax seed oil over the ingredients.

Wash the mint and parsley, pat dry, then finely
chop the leaves. Cut the apricots into small pieces,
then add to the salad along with the herbs and
lentils and mix thoroughly. Season to taste with
salt and pepper.

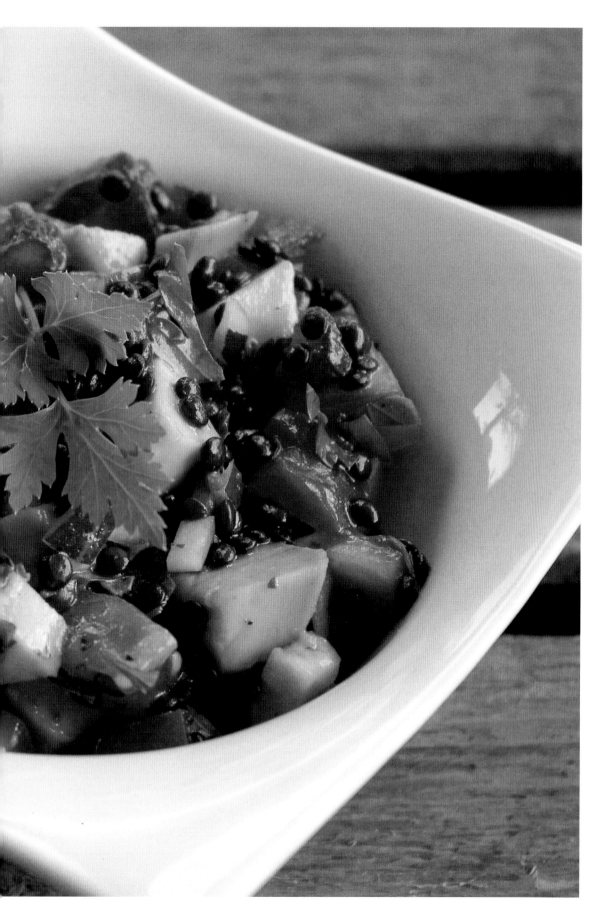

Sicilian bruschetta

Serves 4

300 g honey tomatoes
(or, sweet cocktail
tomatoes)
12 oz/300 g (about
24–30 individual)
small cherry or grape
tomatoes
1 medium, red onion
1 tbsp olive oil
½ tsp sugar
salt, freshly milled
black pepper
juice of 1 lime
12 slices white bread
15 oz/400 g can
chickpeas
fresh basil leaves
fresh Parmesan

Pre-heat the oven to 350 °F (180 °C). Wash and finely dice the tomatoes and place in a bowl. Peel and very finely chop the onion and add to the tomatoes.

Make a marinade by combining the oil, sugar, salt, pepper and lime juice in a small bowl. Pour the marinade over the tomato–onion mixture and leave the flavors to develop for about 20 minutes. Pour off the excess marinade into a bowl.

Arrange the slices of bread on a baking sheet lined with baking paper and toast for a few minutes in the oven until lightly browned.

Rinse and drain the chickpeas under running water, then place them in the reserved tomato marinade for 10 minutes. Drain off the liquid and mix the chickpeas into the chopped tomatoes and onions.

Spread the chickpea topping over the toasted bread and garnish with basil leaves. Sprinkle with grated Parmesan, according to taste.

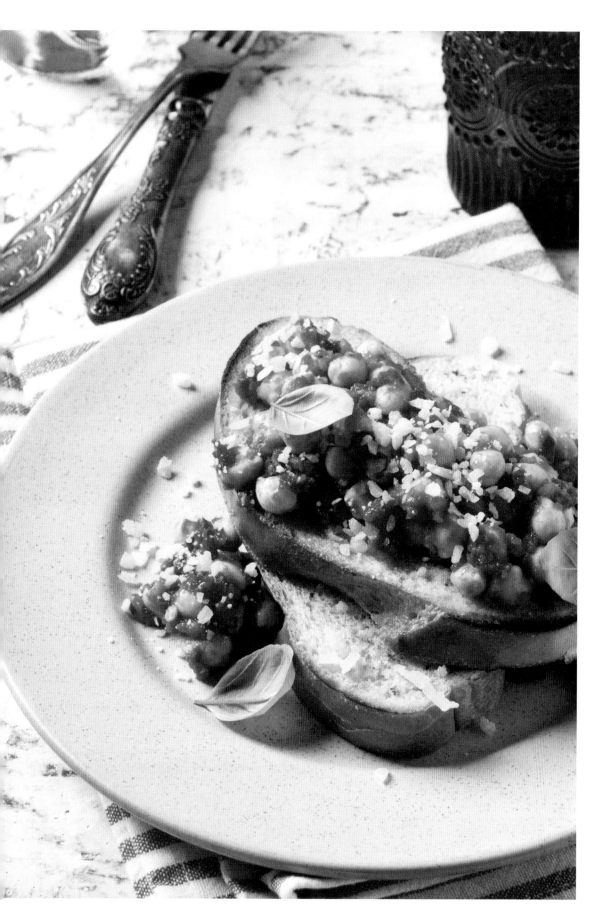

Warm cauliflower salad with peas and feta

Serves 2

½ cauliflower
½ cup/50 g frozen peas
5 oz/150 g feta
½ lemon
½ bunch parsley
½ bunch basil
2 tbsp/30 g mixed seeds and kernels
2 tbsp avocado oil (or olive oil)

Remove the cauliflower leaves, then clean and wash the cauliflower, dividing it into small florets. Cook the cauliflower florets in boiling water for 7 to 10 minutes, adding the peas to cook with the cauliflower for the final 1 to 2 minutes of cooking time.

Meanwhile, cut the feta into small cubes and squeeze the juice from the half lemon. Wash the parsley and basil, pat dry, then tear off and finely chop the leaves. Lightly brown the seeds and kernels for a few minutes in a dry skillet.

Tip the cauliflower and peas into a colander and drain well. Transfer the vegetables to a salad bowl. Add the lemon juice, herbs, toasted mixed seeds, and oil and mix all the ingredients together. Season to taste with salt and pepper. Serve warm.

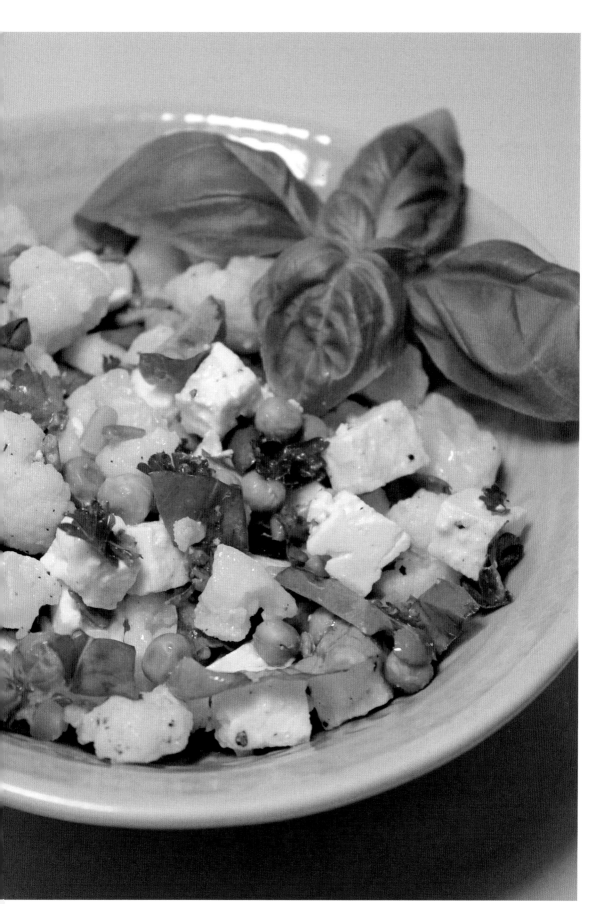

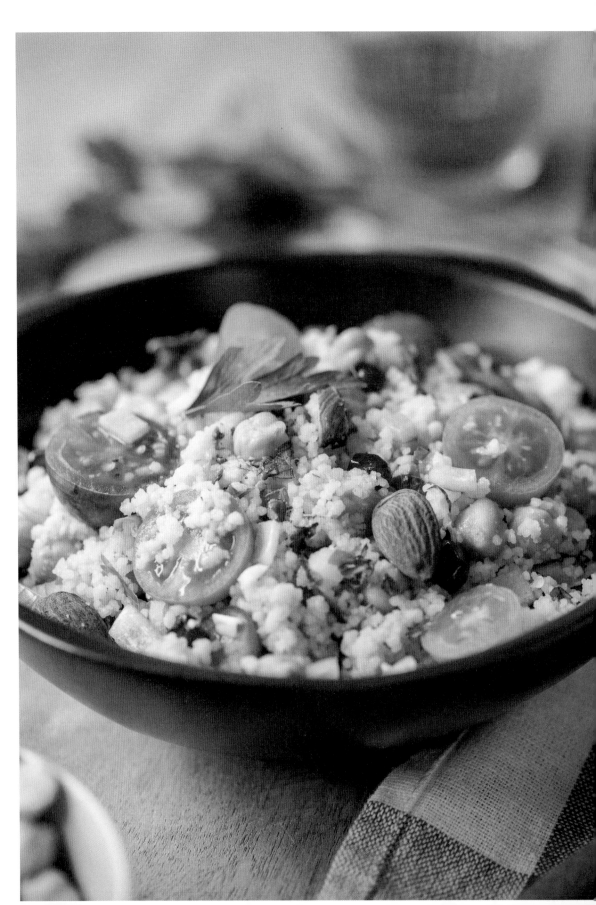

Couscous with pomegranates and almonds

Serves 4

1 cup/250 ml vegetable stock
1⅔ cups/250 g couscous
15 oz/400 g can chickpeas
1 chile
about 1 cup/100 g cherry tomatoes
1 bunch parsley
4 scallions
3 tbsp olive oil
juice of 2 limes
pinch of garam masala
salt, freshly milled black pepper
sugar
¾ cup/100 g almonds, unpeeled
kernels of ½ pomegranate
cilantro leaves

Bring the vegetable stock to a boil, then remove from the heat. Add the couscous and leave to swell.

Rinse the chickpeas under running water. Wash the chile, then slice thinly into rings.

Wash the tomatoes and cut in half. Wash the parsley, shake dry, and finely chop. Clean the scallions and slice into thin rings.

Make a marinade by blending together the oil, lime juice, garam masala, salt, pepper, and sugar to taste. Add the chile and scallions and stir in the chopped parsley.

Once the couscous has soaked up all the stock, mix it with the chickpeas, tomatoes, almonds, and pomegranate seeds, then stir in the parsley marinade. Add additional seasoning to taste, then serve sprinkled with cilantro leaves.

Mediterranean beans with Parmesan

Serves 4

about 3–4 /300 g
medium-sized, waxy
potatoes
1½ cups/300 g fresh,
green beans
1 garlic clove
1 tsp sweet mustard
3 tbsp olive oil
2 tbsp white balsamic
vinegar
salt, freshly milled
black pepper
pinch of garam masala
½ bunch arugula
1 bunch parsley
3½ oz/100 g fresh
Parmesan

Scrub the potatoes and cook in plenty of boiling, salted water.

Wash and clean the beans, then simmer in salted water for about 5 minutes. Drain the beans, then set aside to cool. Peel the garlic, remove the green core and chop very finely. Blend together the garlic, mustard, oil, vinegar, salt and pepper to taste, to make a creamy marinade.

Cut the cooled, cooked potatoes into quarters and mix with the beans in a large bowl. Add the marinade, thoroughly blend all the ingredients together and season with garam masala.

Wash the arugula and tear into small pieces. Wash the parsley, shake dry, and chop very finely. Mix the arugula and parsley into the salad just before serving.

Top the salad with a garnish of Parmesan shavings.

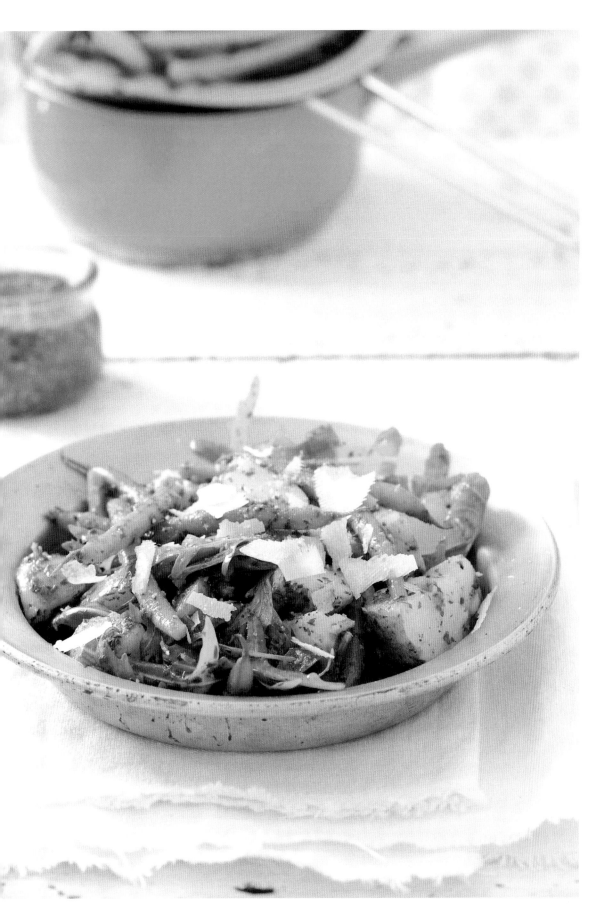

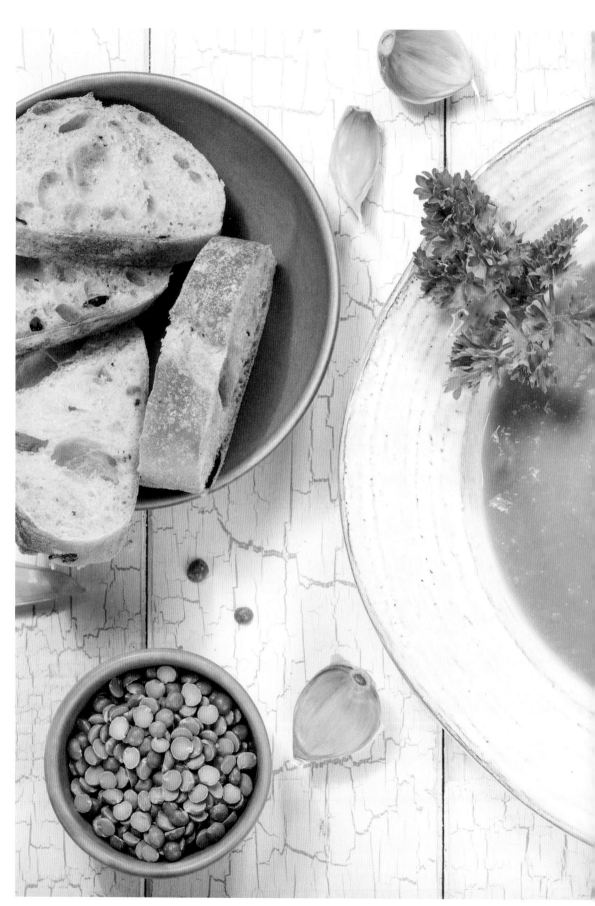

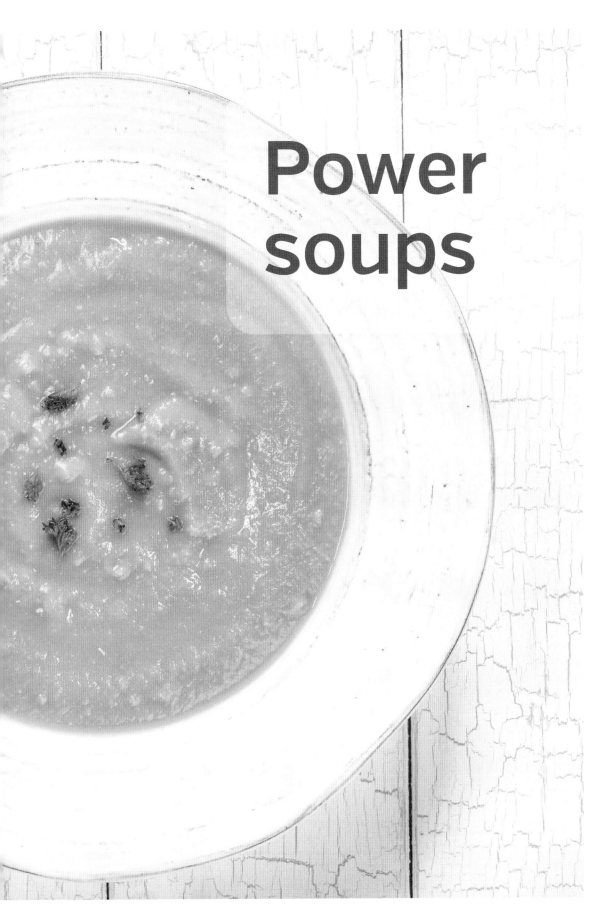

Power soups

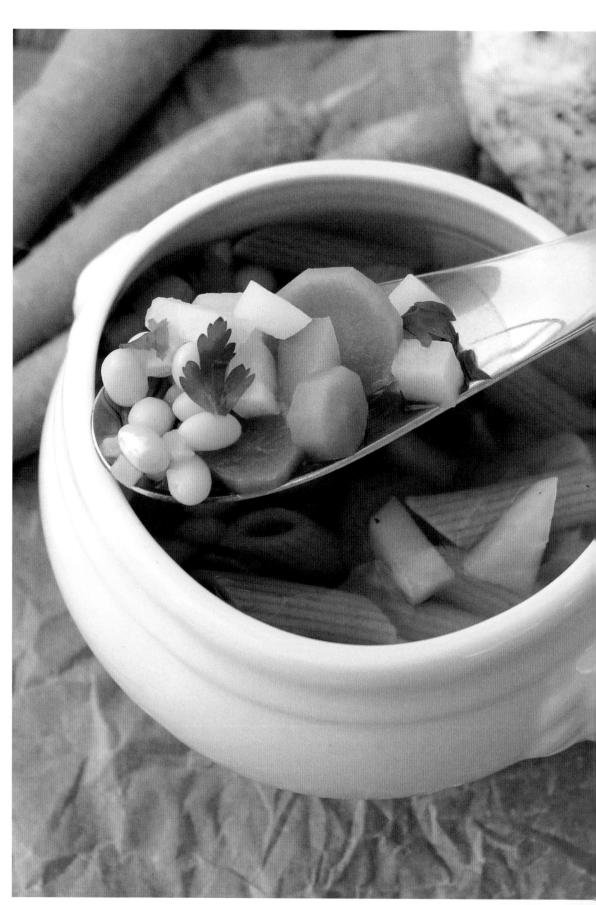

White bean soup with wholegrain pasta

Serves 2

½ cup/100 g dried,
white beans
2 cups/500 ml
vegetable stock
1 onion
1 carrot
about 8 oz/200 g
celery root (celeriac)
1 cup/100 g wholegrain
pasta (penne, fusilli)
2 sprigs parsley
2 tbsp olive oil
salt
freshly milled black
pepper

Soak the beans overnight in water. Next day, drain the beans in a sieve, then place in a saucepan with the vegetable stock and bring to a boil. Simmer for 60 minutes over a low heat.

Peel and finely dice the onion. Peel, rinse, and dice the carrot and celery root. Forty minutes into the beans' cooking time, add the onion, celery root, and carrot to the saucepan and continue to cook. After a further 10 minutes, add the pasta and, if necessary, top up with a little hot water.

Wash the parsley, pat dry, strip off and finely chop the leaves before adding to the saucepan. Stir the olive oil into the soup and season to taste with salt and pepper.

Oriental pumpkin soup

Serves 2

12 oz wedge/300 g
Hokkaido pumpkin
about 1 large/200 g
potatoes
⅓ cup/50 g red lentils
1 onion
1 garlic clove
1–2 tbsp olive oil
2½ cups/600 ml
vegetable stock
saffron, star anise,
according to taste
salt, freshly milled
black pepper
juice of 1 orange
3½ tbsp/50 ml cream

Wash and cut open the pumpkin but do not peel.
Scoop out the seeds using a tablespoon. Weigh
out the required quantity of pumpkin, then cut
into small cubes using a sharp kitchen knife. Peel,
rinse, and dice the potato into small cubes.

Place the lentils in a sieve and rinse in cold water.
Set aside to drain. Peel and finely dice the onion
and garlic.

Heat the olive oil in a saucepan, then add the diced
onion and garlic and sweat for several minutes.
Add the lentils, pumpkin, and potato and pour in
the vegetable stock. Season the soup with saffron,
star anise, salt, and pepper, then cover and simmer
gently for about 20 minutes.

Warm the soup bowls in a low oven. Remove
the star anise from the soup, pour in the orange
juice, then purée the ingredients. Whisk the cream
until stiff, then spoon into a piping bag (or a small
plastic bag with one corner snipped off). Transfer
the soup into the warmed soup bowls and garnish
by quickly piping a whipped-cream heart over the
top.

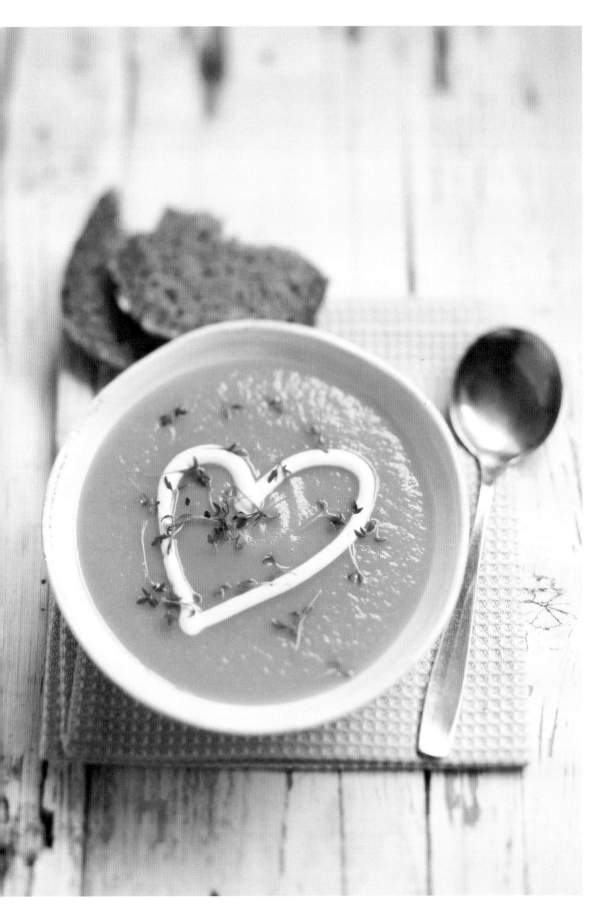

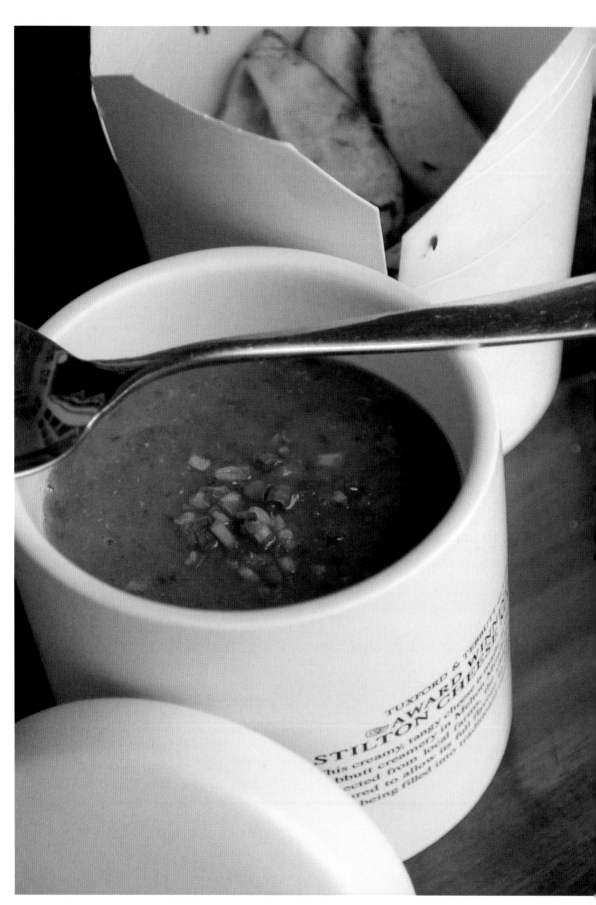

Exotic soup with baked potato wedges

Serves 2

3–4 potatoes
olive oil
1 tsp whole caraway
seeds or rosemary
salt
¼ cup/50 g green or
red lentils
1 onion
1 garlic clove
2–3 medium/100 g
carrots
3 cups/700 ml water
1 ripe banana, sliced
2 tsp turmeric powder
1 tsp curry powder
salt
chives, chopped, or
parsley, finely chopped

Pre-heat the oven to 425 °F (220 °C). Peel the potatoes or, if preferred, scrub clean with a vegetable brush. Cut in half lengthwise and divide into thin wedges. Place in an ovenproof dish and coat thoroughly with olive oil and caraway seeds. Arrange the wedges side by side and bake in the pre-heated oven for about 20 to 30 minutes until the potatoes are lovely and crisp. Sprinkle with salt.

Meanwhile, place the lentils in a sieve, rinse under running water, then set aside to drain. Peel and finely chop the onion and garlic; scrub or peel the carrot and cut into small pieces.

Heat 2 tablespoons of olive oil in a saucepan and sweat the diced onion for a few minutes. Add the carrot, lentils and garlic and sauté gently, stirring frequently. Pour in the water, then add the sliced banana, turmeric, curry powder and salt.

Simmer the soup for 20 to 30 minutes over a gentle heat (check cooking instructions on the packet for the lentils). Season to taste, then purée, if desired. Garnish with chopped chives or parsley.

Miso soup with lentils and pearl barley

Serves 2

2 tbsp pearl barley
2 tbsp green or yellow split peas
3¼ cups/750 ml vegetable stock
½ bell pepper
1 garlic clove
2 tbsp red lentils
2 tbsp peas (fresh or frozen)
about 1 tbsp miso paste
salt, to taste
1–2 tbsp freshly chopped parsley

Rinse the pearl barley and split peas under running water. Cover and cook in the vegetable stock for about 20 minutes.

Wash the bell pepper, remove the seeds and white pith, then cut into tiny pieces. Peel and finely chop the garlic.

Add the bell pepper, garlic and lentils to the pearl barley mixture, then cover and cook for about 10 minutes.

After about 5 minutes, add the peas and cook until tender. Remove the pan from the heat.
Gradually stir in the miso paste, a little at a time, until the desired intensity of flavor is reached.

Season with salt, if required. Serve the soup sprinkled with chopped parsley.

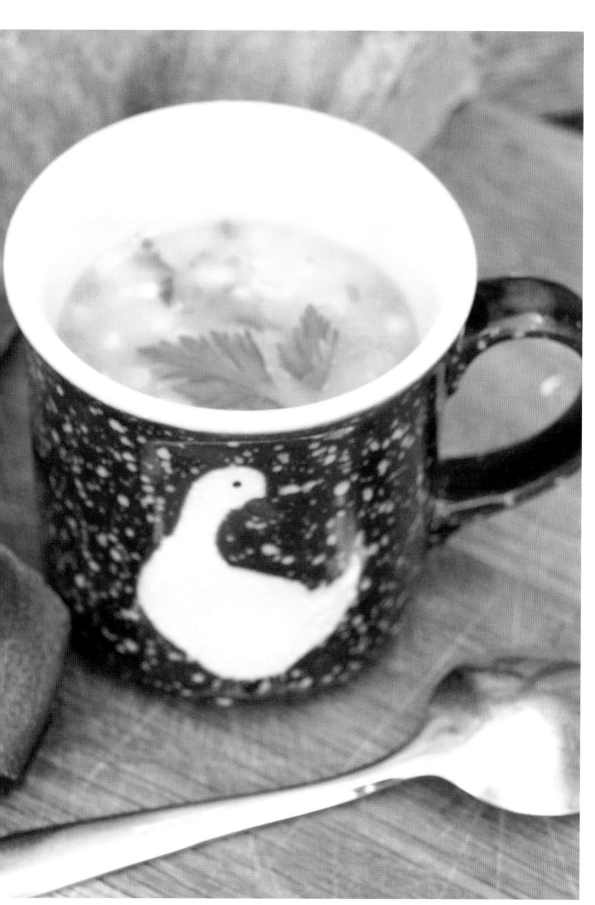

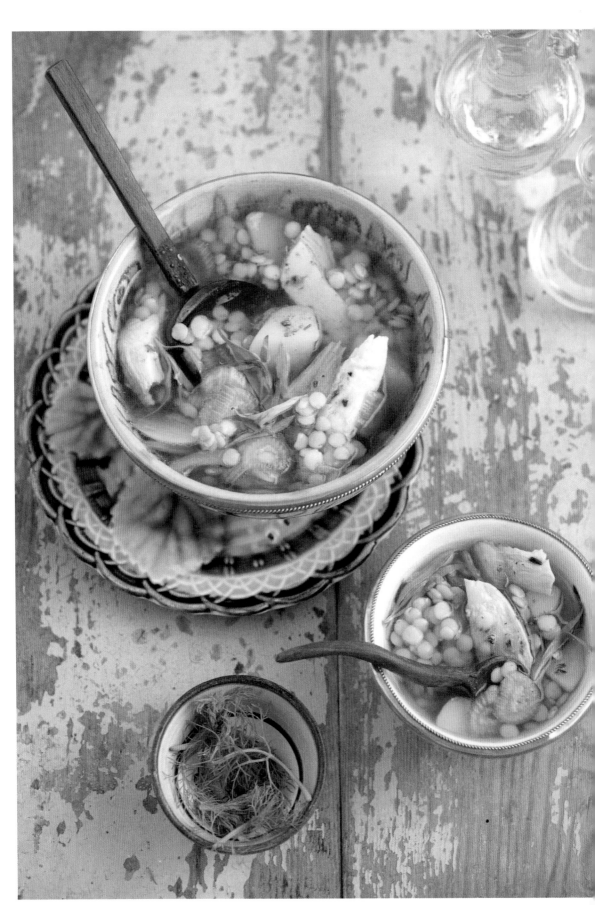

Fennel and lentil soup

Serves 4

3 fennel bulbs
4 sticks celery
1 bunch scallions
4 waxy potatoes
canola or sunflower oil
1 cup/150 g yellow
lentils
½ tsp cumin
½ tsp turmeric
salt, pepper
1 quart/1 liter vegetable
stock
2 chicken breast fillets
1 tbsp soy sauce
juice of 1 lime
bread, to serve

Clean the fennel bulbs and remove what is often a hard, outer layer of skin. Slice each bulb in half, then cut out the stalk, before cutting each half into quarters. Clean the celery sticks, peel ("de-string") and slice into ½-inch/1-cm sections.

Clean the scallions and slice into rings ¾-inch/2-cm thick. Peel and quarter the potatoes.

Heat 3 tablespoons of oil in a large saucepan. Gently fry the lentils in the hot oil until translucent, then add the vegetables, spices, salt, and pepper. Continue to cook the ingredients gently for a little while longer, then pour in the stock and simmer for about 20 minutes.

Heat a little oil in a skillet. Cut each chicken breast into ½-inch/1-cm chunks and sauté in the hot oil. Pour in the soy sauce and continue to cook to reduce the liquid. Remove from the heat after about 5 minutes, season with salt and drizzle with lime juice.

Remove the soup from the heat after about 20 minutes and season to taste with lime juice, salt and pepper. Add the chicken breast chunks to the soup and serve with white bread.

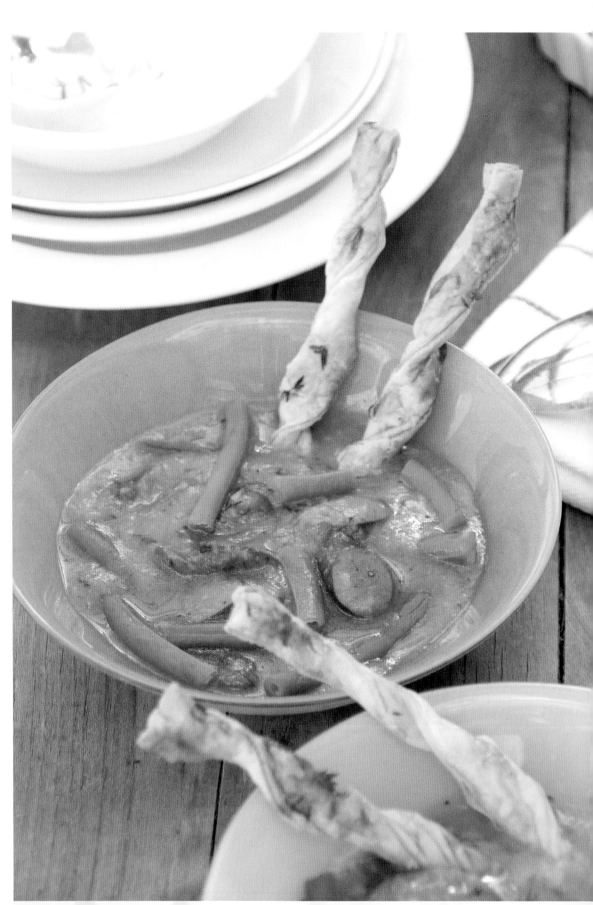

Bean soup with sunchokes and spicy sausage

Serves 2

7 oz/200 g sunchokes
(a.k.a. Jerusalem
artichokes)
1 small onion
2 cups/200 g green
beans
1 tbsp butter
2 cups/500 ml water,
vegetable or beef stock
2 allspice berries or
allspice powder
savory
salt
1–2 pairs of small
sausages (e.g.
frankfurters, cabanossi,
or debrecener)

Peel the sunchokes, rinse, and cut into small pieces. Peel and finely chop the onion. Top and tail the green beans, rinse, then cut in half or into three, depending on how long they are. Cook in a saucepan of boiling, salted water for about 20 minutes until firm to the bite. Drain and set aside.

Melt the butter in a saucepan and sweat the onion. Add the sunchokes and brown for a few minutes over a medium heat, stirring constantly. Pour in the water, season with allspice, savory, and salt, then cover and simmer over a gentle heat for 20 minutes.

Remove the allspice berries, if used whole, and purée the soup. Using a sharp knife, slice the sausages into small pieces and add to the soup along with the cooked beans. Heat for a few minutes, season to taste and serve.

Bean soup with sage and arugula

Serves 2

½ cup/100 g dried, fava
beans
10 small sage leaves
1 leek
2 garlic cloves
4 oz piece/50 g
smoked bacon
1 potato
1 tomato
1⅔ cups/400 ml beef
stock
salt
several arugula leaves
or nasturtium flowers

Wash the fava beans and leave to soak overnight
in plenty of water. Drain and cook in fresh boiling
water for 50 minutes until tender, then drain and
set aside.

Finely chop the sage leaves. Clean the leek and cut
into about ½-inch/1-cm sections. Peel and finely
chop the garlic cloves. Trim any fat off the bacon,
then chop the bacon and fat separately into small
pieces.

Peel and finely dice the potato. Skin the tomato, cut
out the core, and cut the flesh into small pieces.

Slowly melt the bacon fat in a saucepan, then sweat
the leek and garlic in the melted fat. Add the potato,
tomato, and remaining chopped bacon, fry all the
ingredients gently for a few minutes, then pour in
the beef stock.

Add the beans and sage leaves. Cover and simmer
the soup gently for about 20 minutes until the
vegetables are tender. Season to taste. Serve
garnished with arugula leaves.

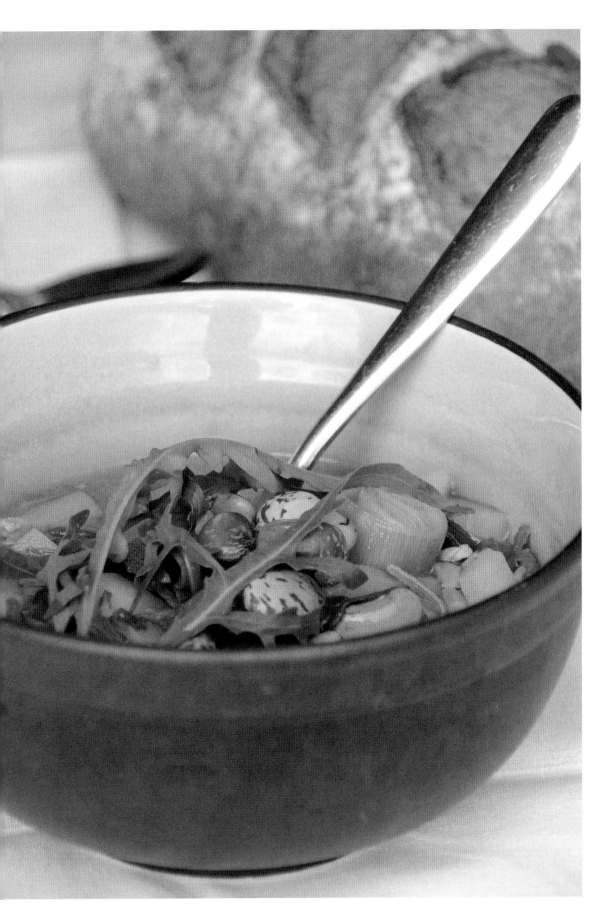

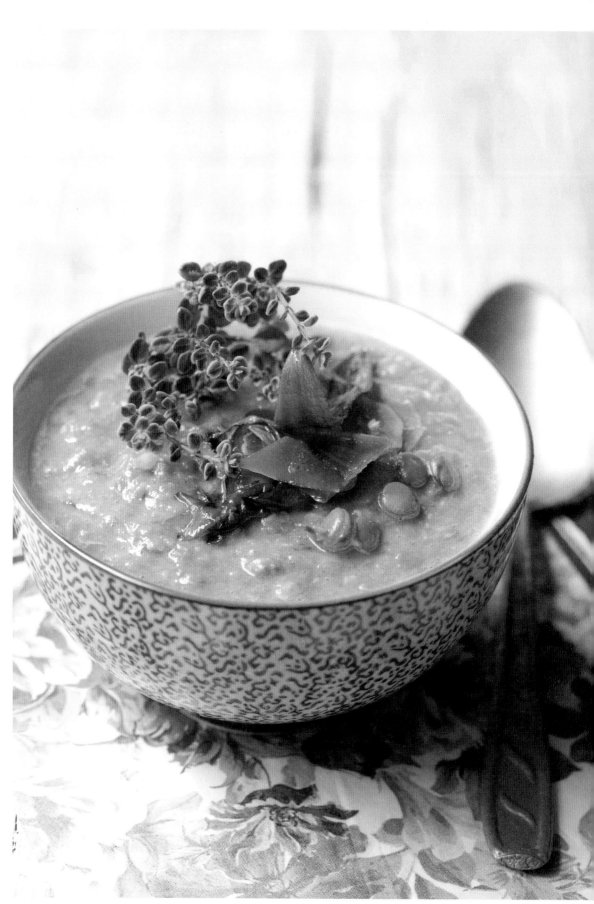

Lentil soup with lemon thyme

Serves 2

¾ cup/150 g red lentils
1 red onion
1 tbsp olive or corn oil
1 cup/250 ml apple
juice
1 cup/250 ml vegetable
stock
2 tbsp lemon juice
2 tsp sugar
1 tsp butter
1 small carrot
2 sprigs lemon thyme
salt
freshly milled black
pepper

Place the lentils in a colander, rinse in cold water and drain. Peel the onion, cut into four, reserve one segment for the garnish, and finely dice the rest.

Heat the oil in a saucepan, then gently sauté the diced onion for a few minutes. Add the lentils and pour in the apple juice and vegetable stock.

Cover and simmer for 10 to 20 minutes until the lentils reach the desired consistency. Season to taste with salt, pepper, a little lemon juice, and 1 teaspoon of the sugar.

For the garnish, peel the carrot, grate into thin slices and sauté with the reserved onion quarter. Garnish with a topping of sliced carrots, onion, and a sprig of lemon thyme.

Pea soup with green curry

Serves 4

2 shallots
2 tbsp olive oil
2 tsp green curry paste
1 quart/1 liter vegetable
stock
3¾ cups/500 g frozen
peas
bunch of fresh mint
½ cup/100 g heavy or
whipping cream
salt, and freshly milled
black pepper

Peel and finely dice the shallots, then sweat in the oil until translucent. Stir in the curry paste and continue to brown for a few minutes before adding the stock. Cook gently for another 5 minutes.

Add the peas, then simmer for a further 5–6 minutes. Wash the mint, shake dry, and roughly chop. Add to the soup, then, using a hand-held processor, purée all the ingredients until absolutely smooth.

Strain the soup through a fine sieve, thoroughly pressing as much liquid as possible out of the residue. Stir in the cream and season to taste with salt and pepper.

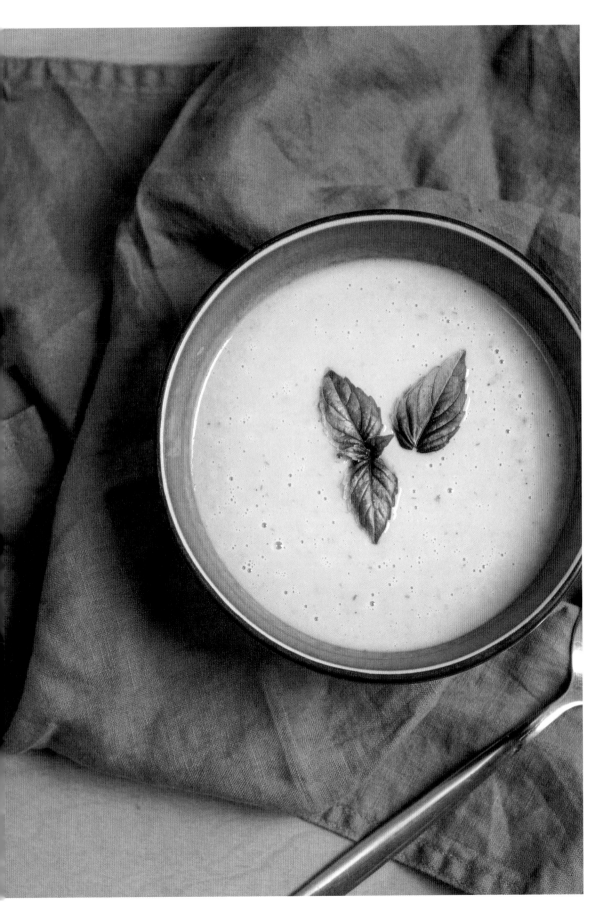

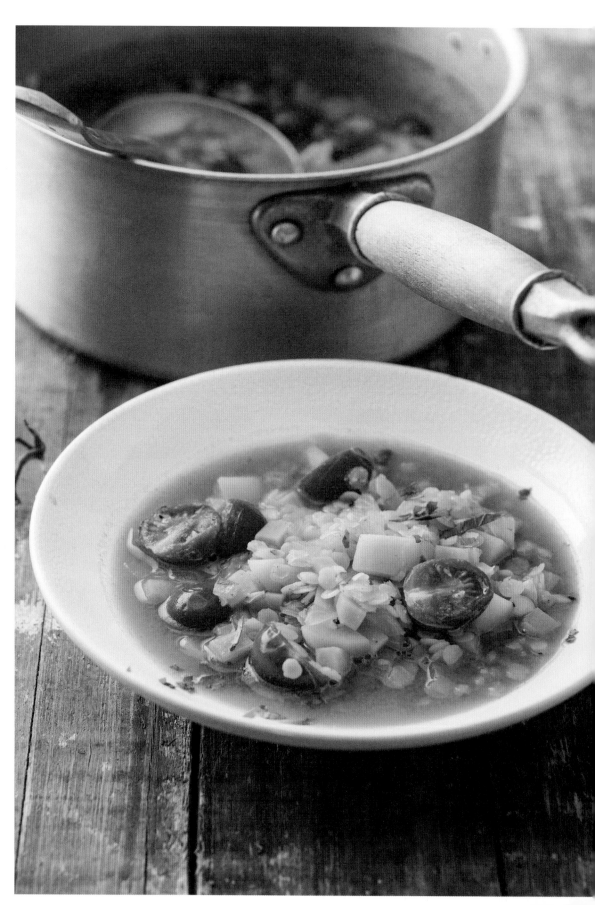

Yellow lentil soup with coconut milk

Serves 2

1 onion
2 garlic cloves
½ chile, depending on taste
2 medium potatoes
1 tbsp olive oil
¼ cup/50 g red lentils
2¾ cups/650 ml water
⅓ inch/1 cm gingerroot
½ tsp coriander seeds
½ tsp ground cumin
1 tsp turmeric powder
salt
4 cherry tomatoes
½ cup/100 ml coconut milk
1–2 cilantro stems, depending on taste

Peel and finely dice the onion. Peel and finely chop the garlic cloves. Wash the chile, cut in half lengthwise, and slice thinly into rings. Peel and finely dice the potatoes.

Heat the olive oil in a saucepan, then brown the onion, garlic, and chile. Rinse the lentils in a sieve under running water, drain, then add to the saucepan along with the diced potatoes. Pour in the water and stir well.

Peel and either finely grate or chop the ginger. Crush the coriander seeds in a pestle and mortar, then add both ingredients, along with the cumin, turmeric, and salt, to taste, to the soup. Cover and simmer for a few minutes until the potatoes and lentils are tender.

Wash and quarter the tomatoes, then add them to the soup.

Add the coconut milk and finely chopped cilantro leaves. Cover the saucepan and continue to heat gently over a low heat for a few minutes.

Crisphead lettuce soup with mint

Serves 2

1 small onion
1 garlic clove
1 large potato
1 tbsp butter
1⅔ cups/400 ml
vegetable stock
⅓ cup/70 g crisphead
lettuce leaves
½ cup/40 g peas (fresh
or frozen)
5 mint leaves
1–2 tbsp whipping
cream
salt

Peel and finely dice the onion and garlic. Peel the potato, rinse briefly, then finely dice.

Melt the butter in a saucepan, add the onion and garlic and sweat until translucent.

Add the diced potato, then pour in the vegetable stock. Season to taste with salt, cover and leave to simmer gently for about 15 minutes.

Wash the lettuce, spin dry, and cut into narrow strips. Add the lettuce and peas to the soup and bring to a boil briefly. Wash the mint leaves, pat dry, and stir into the soup.

Blend in the cream, then, using a hand-held processor, purée all the ingredients until the desired consistency is reached. Season to taste and serve.

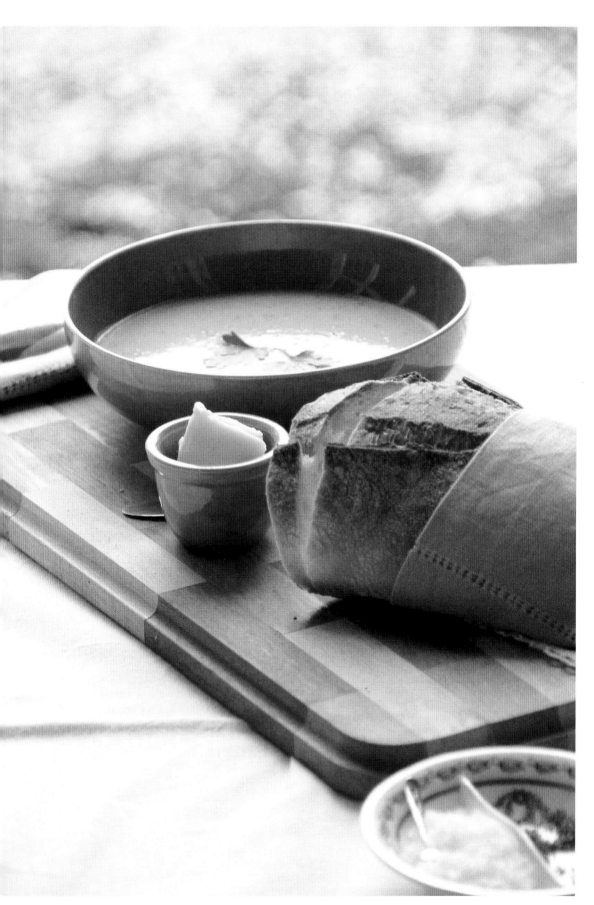

High-energy pea smoothie

Makes 2 glasses

2 scallions
1 parsley stem
handful of sorrel
8 oz/250 g cucumber
1 cup/130 g fresh peas,
shelled
juice and grated peel
of 1 lime
1 cup/250 ml water
salt, freshly milled
black pepper

Clean and roughly chop the scallions. Wash the parsley and sorrel, and shake dry. Wash and roughly chop the cucumber.

Purée the chopped cucumber in a processor along with the herbs, scallions, peas, lime juice, zest, and water. Season to taste with salt and pepper.

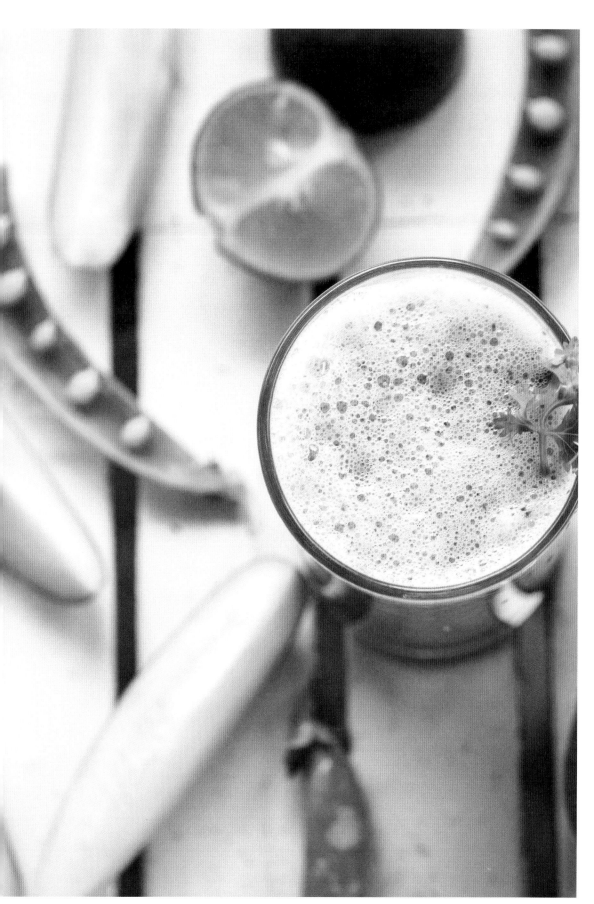

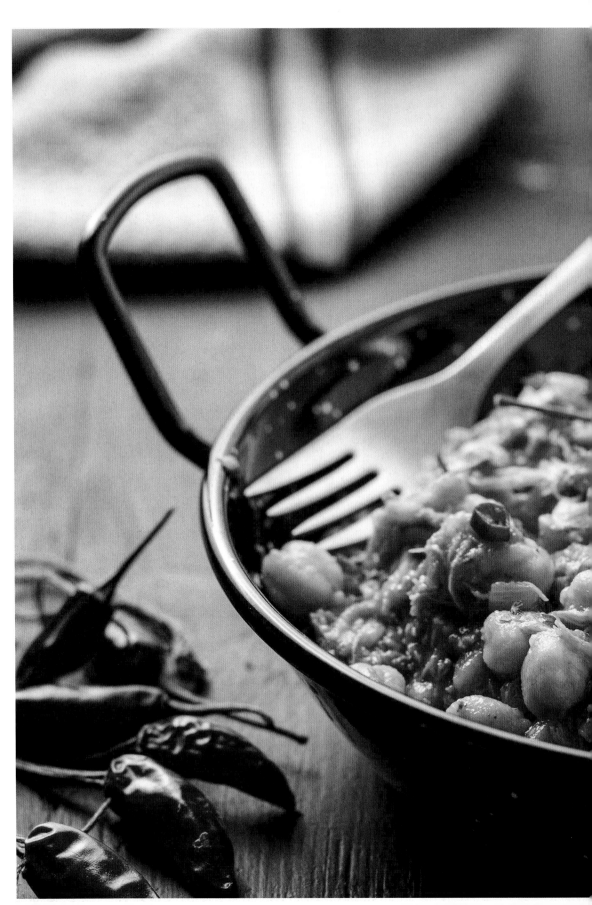

Mediterranean & curry dishes

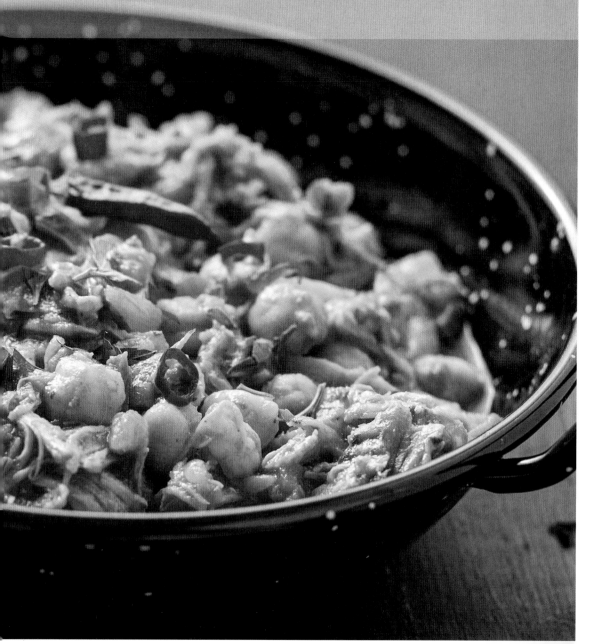

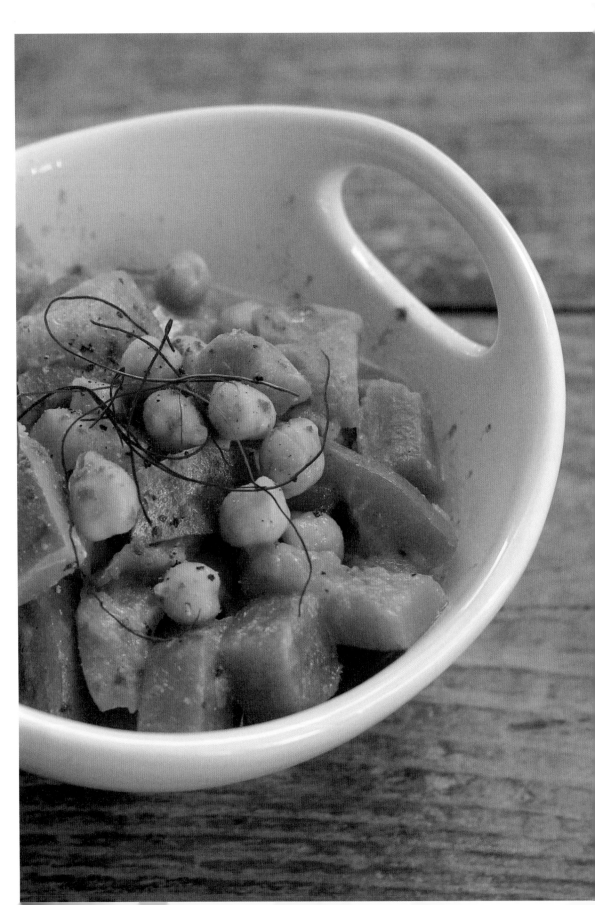

Coconut and chickpea curry

Serves 2

3 tbsp/40 g dried
chickpeas
1 sweet potato
½ Hokkaido pumpkin
(about 8 oz/250 g)
¾ inch/2 cm fresh
gingerroot
2 tbsp coconut oil
1¾ cups/400 ml
coconut milk
1 tsp curry powder
salt
freshly milled black
pepper
red chile threads

Soak the chickpeas overnight in plenty of water. Drain in a sieve, rinse, then place in a saucepan and cover with fresh water. Bring to a boil, cover, and cook for about 40 minutes, then drain.

Peel, wash, and dice the sweet potato. Wash the pumpkin, cut in half, and scoop out the seeds using a tablespoon. Dice the unpeeled pumpkin into cubes. Peel, and finely grate or chop the ginger.

Heat the oil in a skillet. Quickly brown the gingerroot, chickpeas, sweet potato, and pumpkin, stirring occasionally. Pour the coconut milk over the vegetables, cover, and simmer for about 15 minutes. Season with curry powder, salt, and pepper to taste. Transfer the curry to two bowls and garnish with chile threads.

Summer curry with cauliflower and bulgur wheat

Serves 2

1 small onion
⅓ inch/1 cm gingerroot
2 garlic cloves
3 cilantro stems
2–3 tbsp olive oil
2 tsp curry powder
1¾ cups/400 ml
coconut milk
1 small cauliflower
¾ cup/100 g peas
(fresh or frozen)
small can baby corn
½ cup/100 g bulgur
wheat
1 sprig of mint
salt

Peel and finely dice the onion, gingerroot, and garlic cloves. Finely chop the cilantro stems. Heat the olive oil in a saucepan, then sweat the cilantro, onion, gingerroot, and garlic. Sprinkle the curry powder over the mixture, then add the coconut milk. Cover and simmer over a low heat.

Split the cauliflower into small florets, rinse and add to the saucepan. Season with salt to taste and continue to cook for about 5 minutes. Remove the pan from the heat, then add the peas and baby corn. Cover and leave to stand for a few minutes.

Wash the bulgur wheat, place in a bowl, then cover with hot water, according to packet instructions. Mix well, then cover and leave to swell for 5–10 minutes.

Strip the mint leaves from the stalk, wash, and pat dry. Slice into thin strips, mix with the bulgur wheat and season to taste with salt.

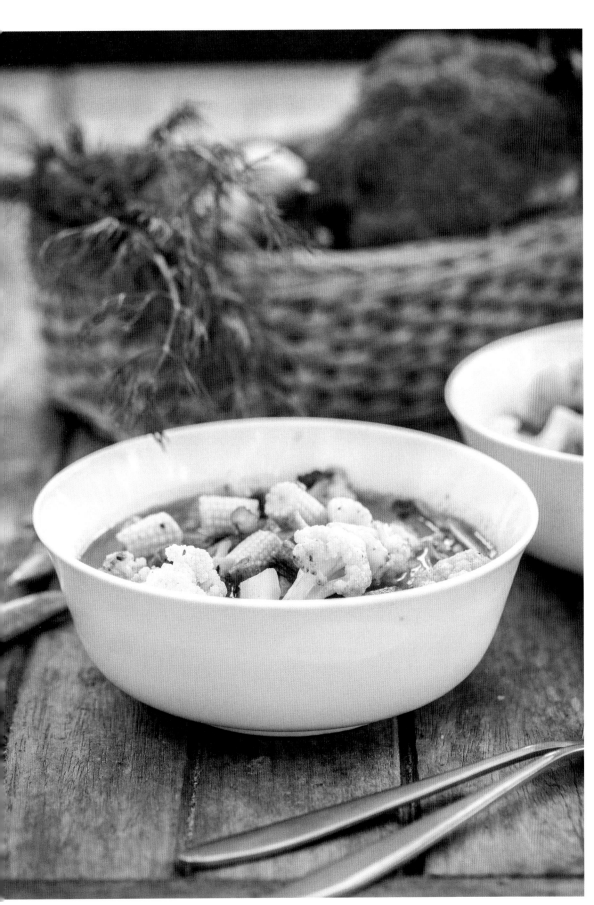

Lentil curry with chickpeas

Serves 4

2 garlic cloves
2 onions
about 1½ inch/4 cm
gingerroot
2 red chiles
5 tbsp oil
1 tsp Madras curry
powder
½ tsp turmeric
½ tsp cumin
pinch of ground
cinnamon
pinch of ground
cardamom
pinch of grated
nutmeg
1 cup/200 g red lentils
15 oz/400 g canned
chickpeas
juice of ½ lime
bunch of cilantro
salt

Peel and finely chop the garlic, onions, and gingerroot. Wash and slice the red chiles into thin rings.

Heat the oil in a deep saucepan and sweat all the above ingredients. Add the curry powder, spices, and salt to taste. Stir in the lentils and cook until translucent.

Cover with warm water, reduce the heat, add a lid and simmer for about 45 minutes. Keep checking that there is still enough liquid in the pan, topping up, if necessary.

Rinse the chickpeas under running water, then add to the lentil mixture after about 15 minutes. Continue to cook until the lentils are tender but still firm to the bite. Add lime juice to taste and more seasoning, if desired.

Wash the cilantro, shake dry, and finely chop. Sprinkle over the curry before serving.

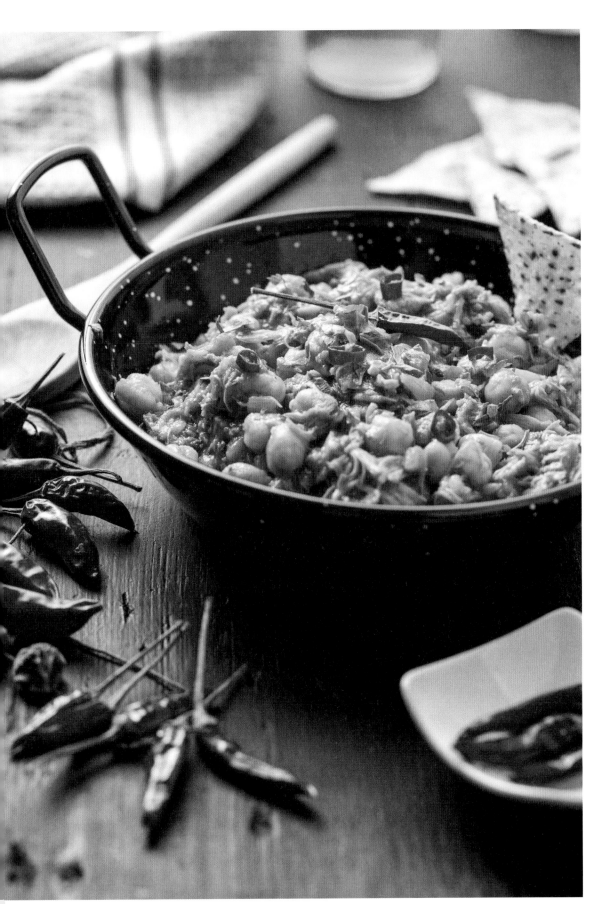

Curry with eggplant, cashew nuts, and chickpeas

Serves 2

2½ cups/400 g
cooked chickpeas
(1 cup/175-190 g dry
weight), or canned
1 eggplant
1 small zucchini
1 yellow bell pepper
1 onion
2 garlic cloves
1 tbsp cashew nuts
1 chile
4 tbsp olive oil
curry powder
cumin powder
salt
1⅔ cups/400 ml water
or vegetable stock
fresh cilantro or
parsley

Rinse and drain the canned chickpeas.

Wash the eggplant and zucchini, cut off the stalks, and dice. Wash the bell pepper, cut into four lengthwise, remove the stalk, seeds, and white pith, then cut into small pieces. Peel and finely dice the onion and garlic. Toast the cashew nuts in a fat-free, non-stick skillet.

Wash the chile, cut in half, discard the seeds, and slice into thin rings. Heat the olive oil in a skillet, then sweat the onions and garlic. Add the bell pepper, eggplant and zucchini, then brown on all sides over a medium heat, stirring occasionally.

Add the chickpeas. Season to taste with curry, cumin, and salt. Add the sliced chile and top up with enough water to cover all the ingredients.

Cover and simmer the curry for 20 minutes. Wash the cilantro, pat dry, and finely chop. Just before serving, stir the cilantro into the curry and season to taste.

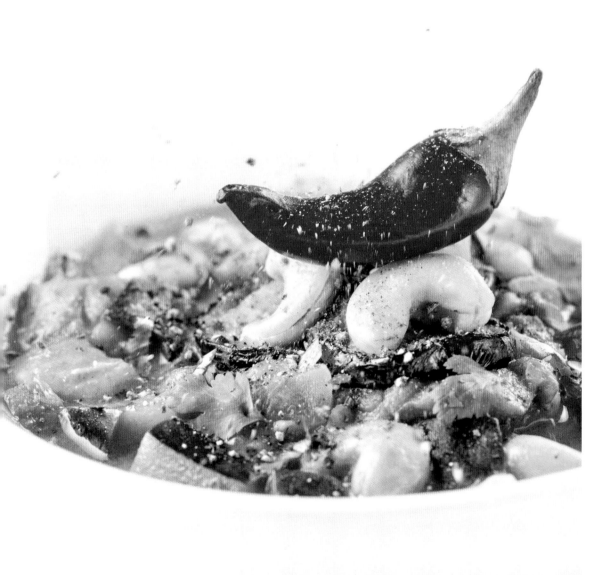

Lentil curry with cucumber yogurt

Serves 4

6 tbsp oil
¾ cup/150 g red lentils
¾ cup/150 g yellow
lentils
2 cups/500 ml
vegetable stock, salted
juice of ½ lime
1 large onion
1 bell pepper
1 zucchini
1 chile
1 tsp sugar
¼ tsp turmeric
1 tsp yellow or Madras
curry powder
1 cup/7–8 oz canned
tomatoes, chopped
½ bunch each of
parsley and cilantro
salt

For the dip
½ cucumber
1½ cups/300 g Greek-
style yogurt
¼ tsp salt

Heat 3 tablespoons of the oil in a deep saucepan. Add the red and yellow lentils to the hot oil and fry gently until translucent, stirring constantly. Pour in the stock and lime juice, season with salt to taste, cover, and simmer over a low heat.

Peel and finely dice the onion. Wash, seed and finely dice the bell pepper. Wash and finely dice the zucchini. Slice the chile pepper into thin rings.

Heat the remaining oil in a large skillet, then brown the chopped onion, zucchini, bell pepper and chile. Sprinkle with the sugar, then cook until the vegetables begin to caramelize. Add the turmeric and curry powder, stirring constantly.

Blend in the tomatoes, season with salt and simmer gently to amalgamate. Add the cooked lentils and add more seasoning if necessary.

Wash the parsley and cilantro, shake dry, then chop and sprinkle over the curry to serve.

To make the dip, combine the yogurt and salt. Peel, seed and finely chop the cucumber. Mix with the yogurt and serve as an accompaniment to the curry.

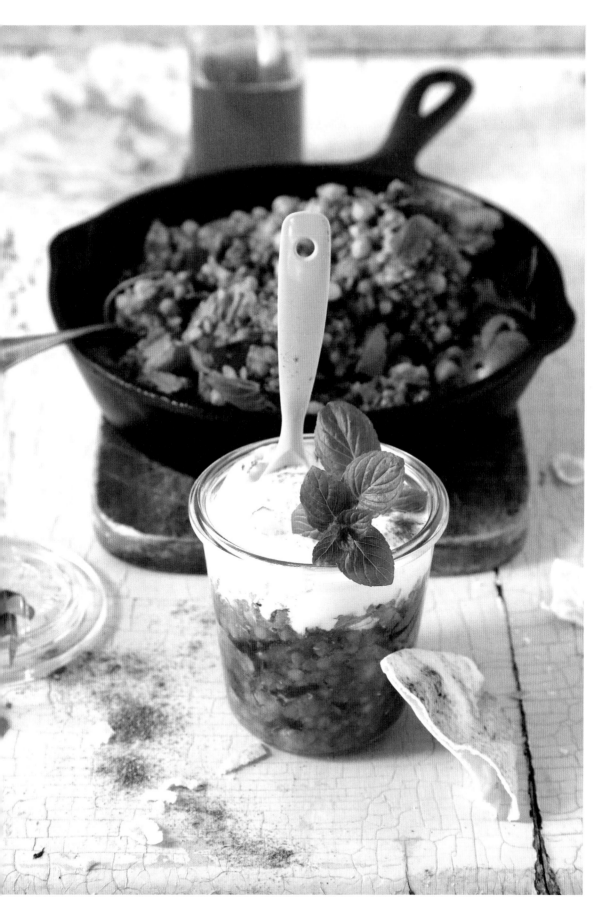

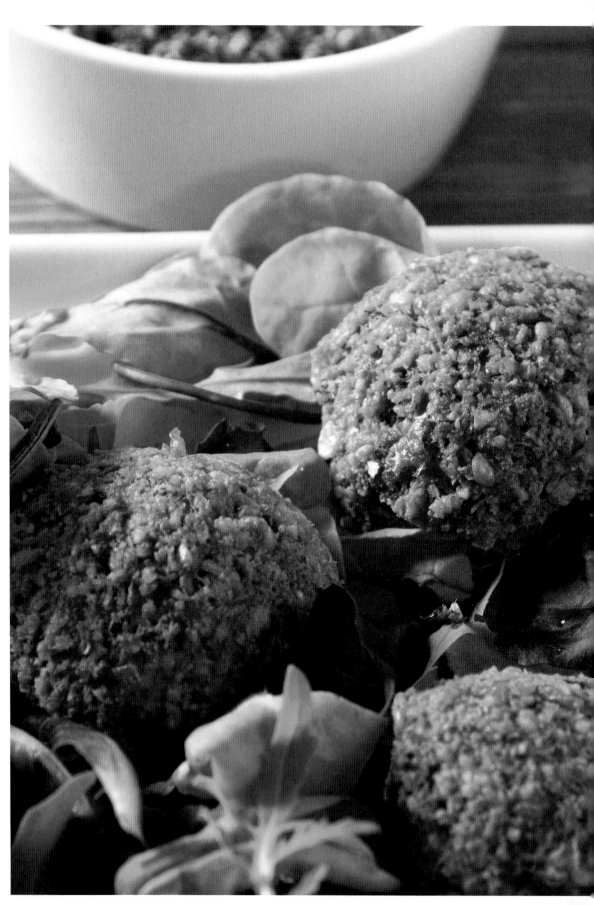

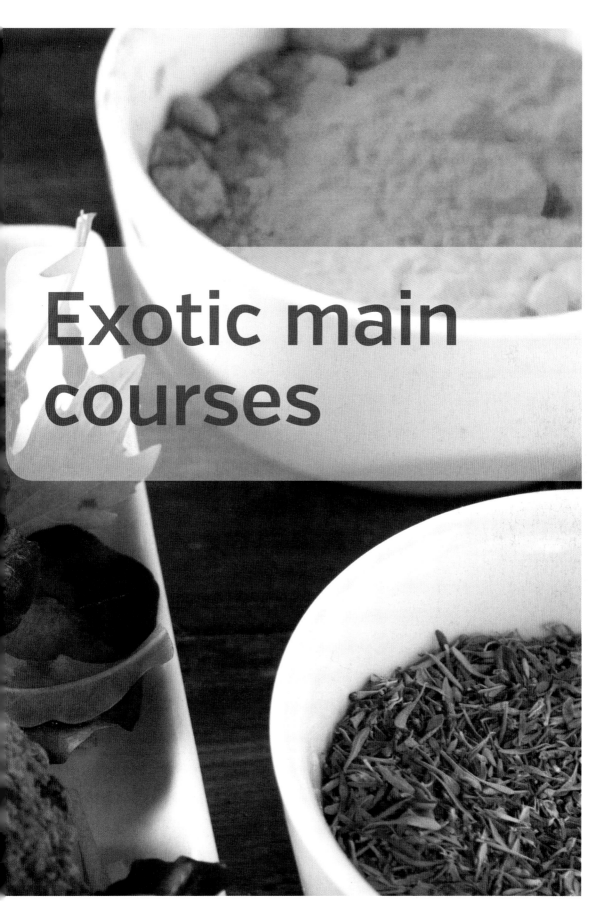

Exotic main courses

Dal with kidney beans

Serves 4

¾ inch/2 cm fresh
gingerroot
3 garlic cloves
1 onion
2 chiles
1 x 14 oz/400 g can
kidney beans
4 tbsp oil
½ tsp red curry powder
¼ tsp turmeric
pinch of ground
nutmeg
pinch of ground
cinnamon
salt
½ cup/100 g red lentils
2 cups/500 ml
vegetable stock
tomato paste to taste

Peel and finely chop the gingerroot and garlic cloves. Peel the onion and slice into thin rings. Wash the chiles and slice into thin rings.

Rinse and drain the kidney beans in fresh water.

Heat the oil in a skillet, then sweat the gingerroot, garlic, and onion. Add the curry powder, turmeric, nutmeg, cinnamon, sliced chiles, and salt to taste, stirring frequently. Stir in the lentils and fry until translucent, then add the kidney beans.

Pour in the vegetable stock, then cover and simmer until all the liquid has disappeared. If the liquid has all been absorbed before the lentils are tender, add a little more warm water.

Add more curry seasoning or salt to taste, if desired. If the dal is too salty or spicy, counteract this by blending in some tomato paste.

Serve this dal dish with an accompaniment of yogurt dip (p. 94) and naan or pitta bread.

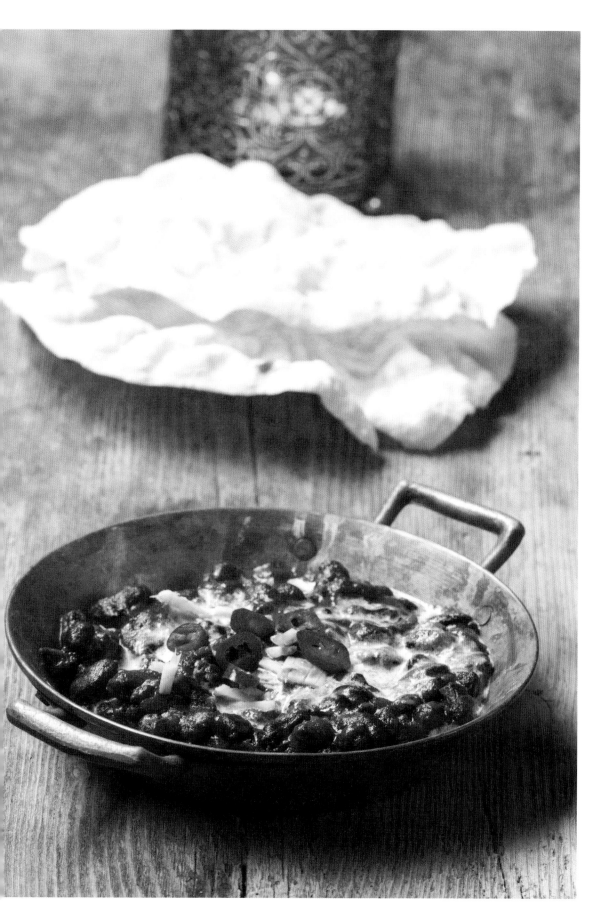

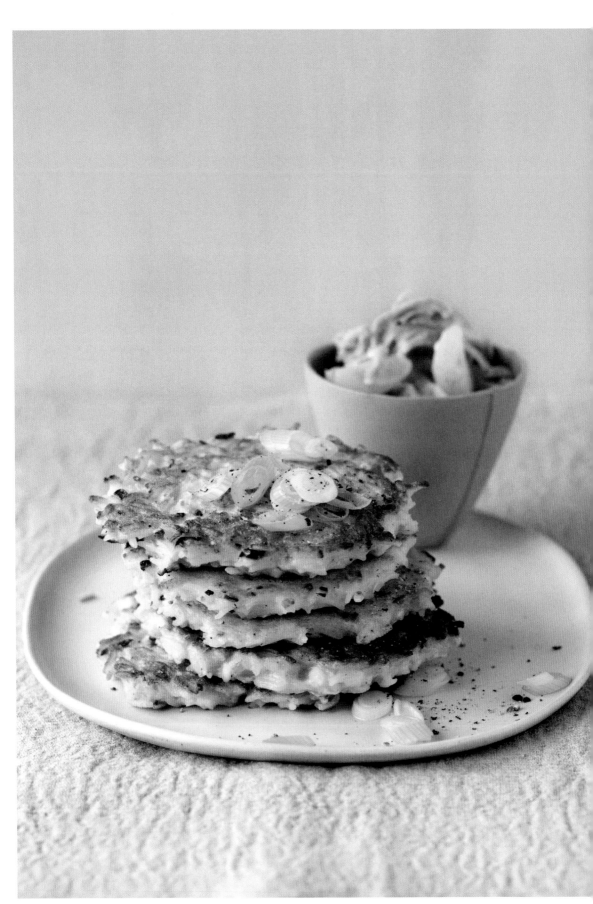

Lentil and rice fritters with winter salad

Makes 8 fritters

For the fritters
6–8 tbsp cooked rice
¼ cup/50 g red or yellow lentils
1 egg
thyme, oregano
salt
freshly milled black pepper
3 tbsp sunflower oil

For the salad
3 carrots
1 medium sweet potato
1 tbsp olive oil
1 tbsp yogurt
juice of 1 lime
salt, sugar

Wash the rice and lentils separately, then cook separately until tender, according to the instructions on the packet. Combine the rice and lentils (in the amounts indicated in the recipe) with the egg, thyme, oregano, salt, and pepper to taste.

Heat the sunflower oil in a skillet. Add one portion of the lentil-and-rice mixture at a time to the skillet, pressing it into a flat round using a fork. When the fritter is crisp on one side, flip it over and brown the other side.

To make the salad, peel the carrots and sweet potato, then roughly grate both ingredients or cut into thin matchsticks.

Blend the oil and yogurt, then mix with the grated vegetables. Season the salad to taste with lime juice, salt, and sugar.

Parsnip chips with lentils and beets

Serves 2

1–2 parsnips
2–3 (about 8 oz/250 g)
beets
1 onion
2 garlic cloves
2–3 sprigs of thyme
1 tbsp grated zest of an
unwaxed lemon
salt
freshly milled black
pepper
3–4 tbsp olive oil
½ cup/100 g lentils
3–4 tbsp vinegar
1–2 tbsp freshly
chopped parsley
small amount of fresh
horseradish

Pre-heat the oven to 400 °F (200 °C). Scrub the parsnips using a vegetable brush, rinse, and shave into thin layers using a potato peeler. Scrub and rinse the beets thoroughly. Leaving on the peel, cut into segments (about ¼ inch/0.5 cm thick). It is advisable to wear disposable rubber gloves for this step to avoid staining.

Peel and slice the onion into rings. Peel the garlic and slice into thin rings or chop finely. Mix the beets, onion, and garlic together in an ovenproof dish, then sprinkle with finely chopped thyme leaves. Top with the parsnip shavings, season with salt and pepper, and drizzle with olive oil. Cook in the oven for about 30 minutes. While the finished parsnip chips should be nice and crisp, they can easily become too dark so, if necessary, turn down the oven temperature to 325 °F (160 °C).

Tip the lentils into a sieve, rinse under running water, then drain. Cook in a saucepan until tender, according to the instructions on the packet, then combine with the vinegar, salt to taste, and parsley. Finally, grate a little horseradish over the beets, according to taste.

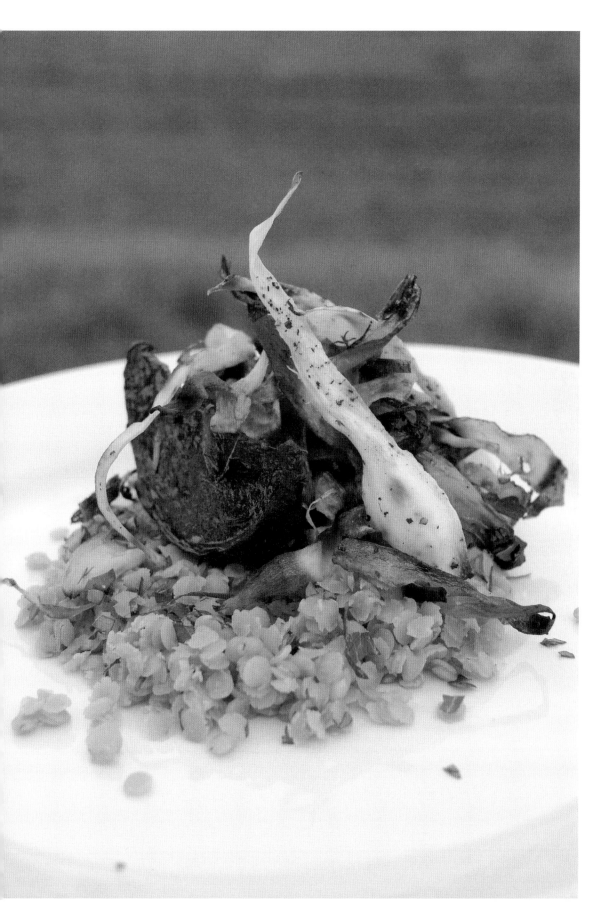

Falafel sticks

Serves 4

1 cup/200 g dried
chickpeas
2 garlic cloves
1 red onion
½ bunch cilantro
1 tsp harissa (Moroccan
spicy paste)
½ tsp cumin
2 tbsp breadcrumbs
1 tbsp sesame seeds
oil, for frying

Soak the chickpeas overnight. Next day, drain and rinse under running water.

Peel the garlic and remove the green core. Peel and dice the onion. Wash the coriander and shake dry.

Place the chickpeas, garlic, onion, cilantro, harissa, and cumin in a mixing bowl, and purée. The mixture should be malleable enough to mold into shape: if it is too soft, knead in some breadcrumbs. If too stiff, add a little more water.

Shape the falafel mixture into sticks and press onto wooden skewers. Combine the breadcrumbs and sesame seeds, then coat the falafel sticks in the breadcrumb mixture.

Pre-heat the oven to 325°F (160 °C). Fry in a deep-fat fryer or heat the oil in a deep saucepan and fry the falafel sticks, a portion at a time, for about 2–3 minutes. Drain on paper towels, then place in the oven to keep warm until they are all fried. Hummus or couscous salad make an excellent accompaniment to falafel sticks.

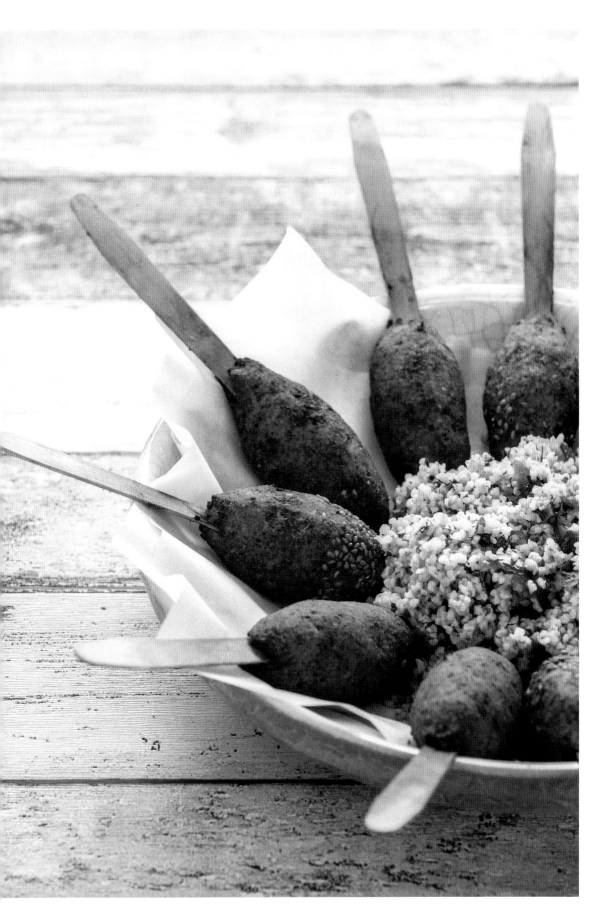

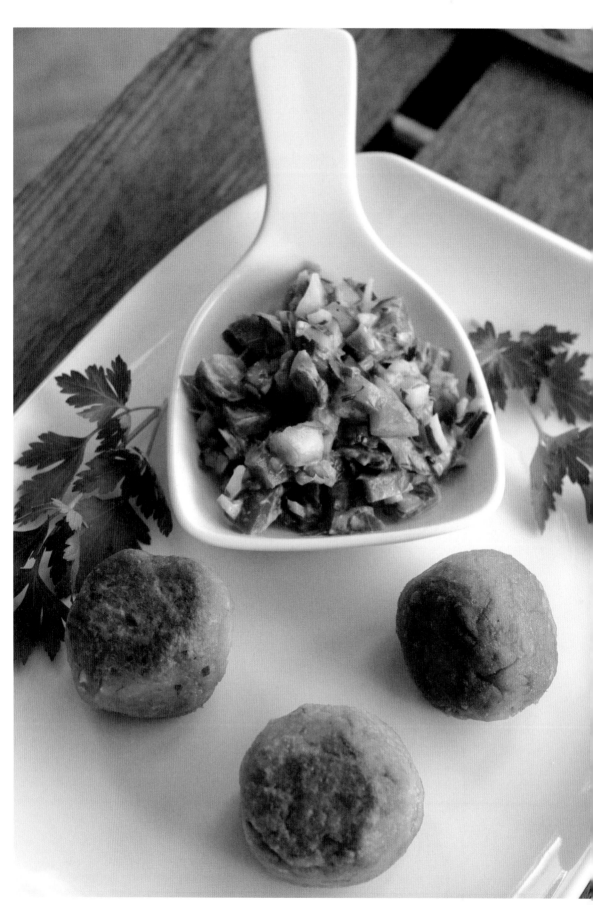

Maca falafels

Makes 8 falafels

6 tbsp/80 g dried
chickpeas
1 small onion
1 garlic clove
½ bunch flat-leaf
parsley
salt
freshly milled black
pepper
1 tsp caraway seeds
1 tbsp Maca powder
1 tsp baking powder
oil, for frying

Soak the chickpeas overnight in plenty of water. Drain in a sieve, then rinse in fresh, running water. Purée to a smooth paste in a hand-held processor or food mixer.

Peel and finely dice the onion. Peel and crush the garlic. Wash the parsley, shake dry and finely chop. Add the parsley, onion, garlic, salt, pepper, caraway seeds, Maca powder, baking powder, and 3½ tablespoons of water to the chickpea purée. Knead the mixture thoroughly by hand. If the dough is too stiff to mold into shape easily, add a little more water. If too soft, mix in a little wholegrain flour. Leave the dough to rest for about 30 minutes.

Shape the chickpea mixture into balls the size of table tennis balls. Heat the oil in a skillet and fry on all sides until golden brown. Drain the falafel on paper towels and serve.

Lentil pilau

Serves 4

1 cup/200 g basmati
rice
½ tsp salt
¼ tsp saffron strands
1 tsp sugar
2 tbsp butter
1 onion
1 leek
6 dried apricots
3 tbsp oil
½ cup/100 g yellow
lentils
salt
pinch of garam masala
about 1 cup/250 ml
warm water
¾ cup/100 g fresh or
frozen peas

Bring the rice to a boil in double the quantity of warm water, season with salt, cover and cook over a low heat. The finished rice should be nice and light when fluffed up with a fork. Pre-heat the oven to 300 °F (150 °C).

Crush the sugar and saffron strands in a pestle and mortar. Melt the butter in a saucepan, add the saffron-and-sugar mixture and let it sweat, stirring constantly, then add the rice. Cover the saucepan with a lid, and place in the pre-heated oven to cook for 20 minutes.

Peel and finely dice the onion. Clean the leek, rinse, and slice into thin rings. Dice the dried apricots.

Heat the oil in a skillet. Add the lentils and sweat, stirring constantly, until translucent. Add the onion, leek, apricots, salt to taste, and garam masala. Pour in the lukewarm water, cover the pan with a lid and bring to a boil, then reduce the heat to a simmer.

After about 20 minutes, add the peas and continue to cook until the liquid has largely evaporated.

Remove the rice from the oven, then mix with the ingredients in the skillet.

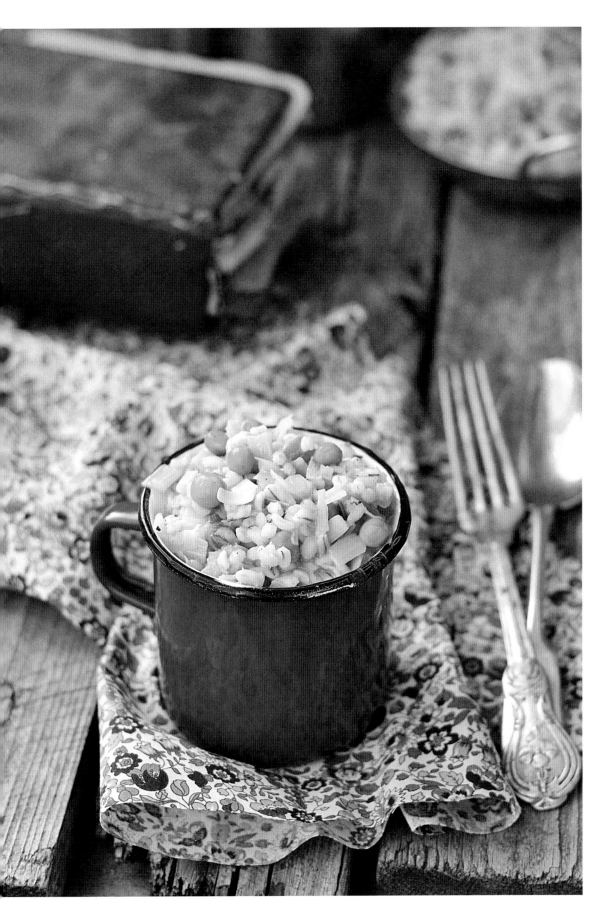

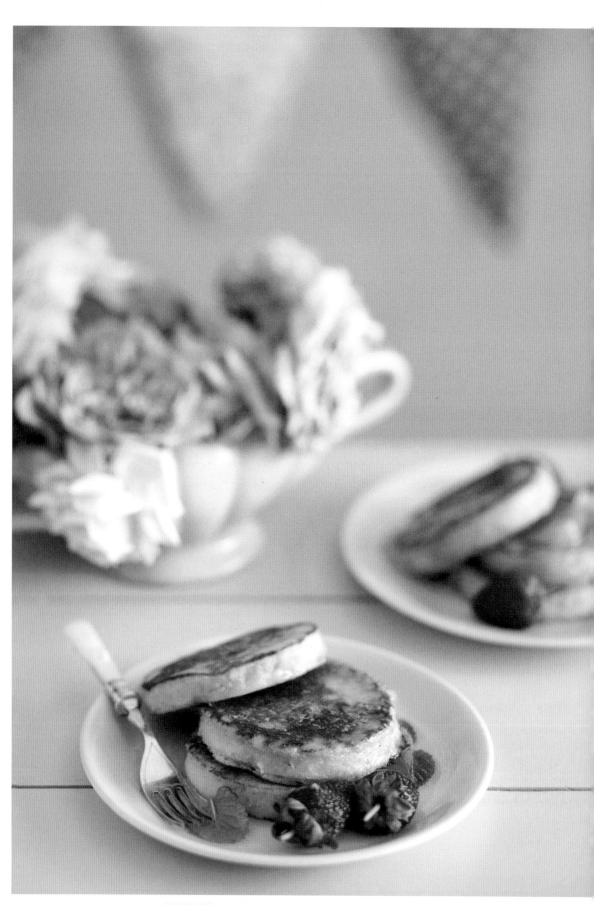

Apple and chickpea pancakes

Serves 8

½ cup/50 g chickpea flour
1 cup/100 g spelt or wholegrain flour
¼ level tsp baking powder
pinch of salt
3 tbsp/40 g raw cane sugar
2 tbsp/30 g sunflower oil
1 apple (about 3½ oz/ 100 g)
coconut or vegetable oil, for frying

Sift the chickpea flour into a large bowl with the spelt flour, baking powder, and salt and mix thoroughly.

Add the raw cane sugar, oil, and 4 tablespoons/ 60 ml of water, then combine the ingredients into a smooth dough, using an electric hand-held mixer.

Wash the apple, wipe dry with a cloth, cut into quarters, and remove the core. Finely grate the apple and stir into the mixture.

Heat a little oil in a non-stick skillet or stainless steel skillet. Add 1 tablespoon of dough to the skillet for each pancake and flatten into a round about ⅓ inch/1 cm thick. Shake gently after about ½ minute to prevent the pancake from sticking. Fry on both sides until golden brown. Drain on paper towels, if necessary, to absorb any excess fat.

Moroccan bean patties

Serves 4

1 x 14 oz/400 g can of
mixed beans
½ bunch parsley
3 scallions
½ tsp cumin
salt, freshly milled
black pepper
2 tbsp flour
1 egg
2 tbsp oil
3 tbsp panko
breadcrumbs

Drain the beans. Wash the parsley and shake dry.
Clean and roughly chop the scallions.

Combine the beans, scallions, parsley, and cumin,
then purée. Do not worry if chunks of beans are
still visible in the resulting mixture.

Season to taste with salt and pepper. Knead the
flour and egg into the mixture and shape into
patties.

Pre-heat the oven to 350 °F (180 °C). Heat the
oil in a skillet. Coat the patties in breadcrumbs,
then fry for about 5 minutes on each side before
finishing off in the oven for a further 10 minutes.

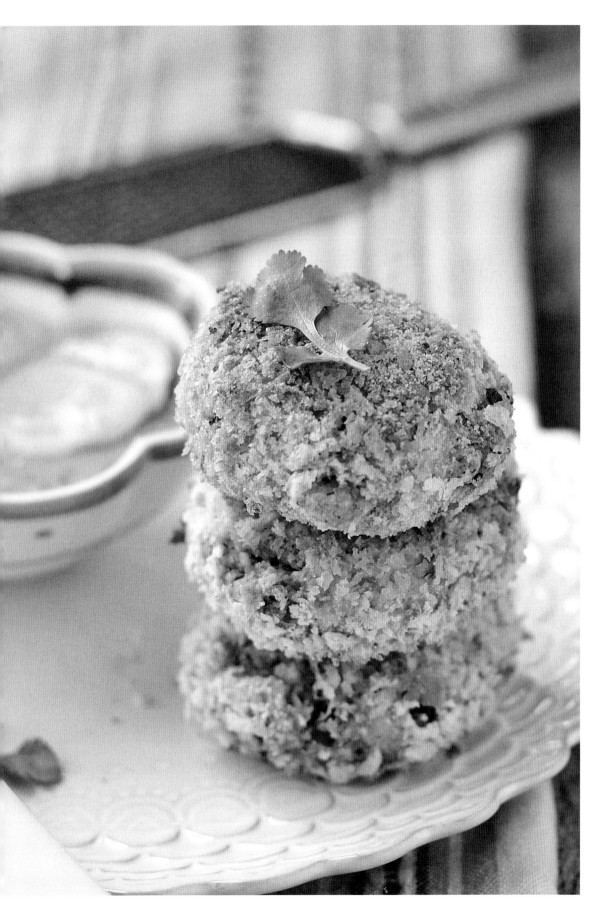

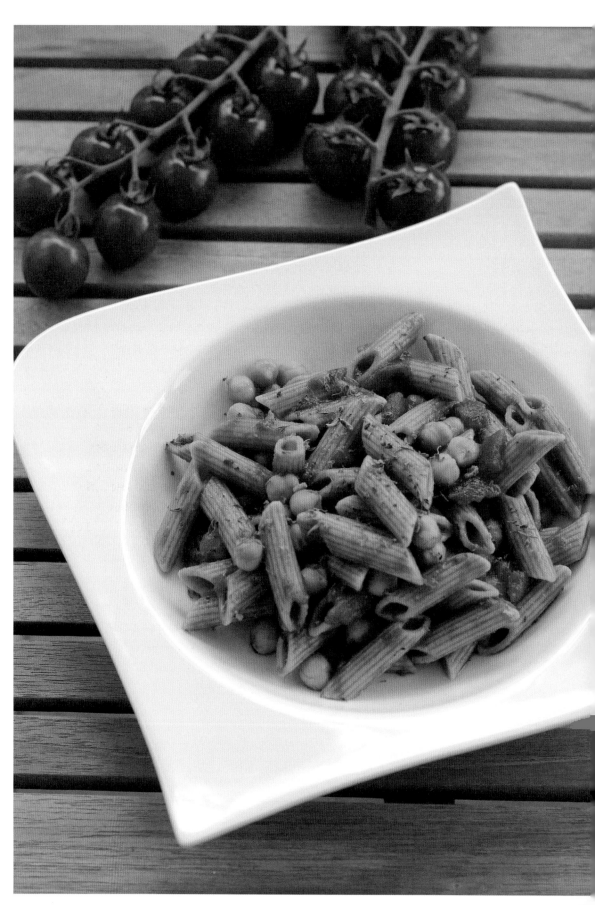

Pasta with chickpeas

Serves 2

½ cup/80 g dried
chickpeas
2¼ cups/250 g
wholegrain spelt pasta
(penne)
1 onion
1 garlic clove
3 medium/400 g
tomatoes
thyme
oregano
1 tbsp olive oil
salt
freshly milled black
pepper

Soak the chickpeas overnight in plenty of water. Drain in a sieve, rinse well and place in a saucepan in plenty of water. Bring to a boil, cover, and simmer over a low heat. Check the chickpeas after 45 minutes to see if they are tender and, if so, drain.

Cook the pasta according to the instructions on the packet, then drain and "shock" the pasta in cold water. Peel and finely chop the onion; peel and crush the garlic clove. Plunge the tomatoes briefly in boiling water. Drain, pierce and peel off the skins, discard the core, and roughly chop. Purée or blend in a processor with ⅔ cup/150 ml of water, then season with thyme and oregano.

Heat the olive oil in a saucepan, and sweat the onion and garlic. Add the chickpeas and chopped tomato, cover, and simmer for 10 minutes. Season to taste with salt and pepper. Add the pasta to the sauce and mix well. Re-heat the ingredients briefly and serve.

Chickpea and narrowleaf plantain medallions

Serves 4

1¼ cups/250 g dried chickpeas
5 bay leaves
½ cup/100 ml vegetable stock
1 tbsp thyme leaves
1 tbsp lovage
20 narrowleaf plantain leaves
small amount of spelt flour
salt, freshly milled black pepper
grated nutmeg, if desired

Soak the chickpeas overnight.

Drain and rinse the chickpeas. Cook with the bay leaves in the vegetable stock until soft. Remove the bay leaves. Chop the lovage and plantain leaves.

Mix the chickpeas with the thyme, lovage, and plantain leaves, then purée and season to taste. Add a little more vegetable stock or spelt flour, as required.

Shape the mixture into small rounds and fry on both sides until golden brown.

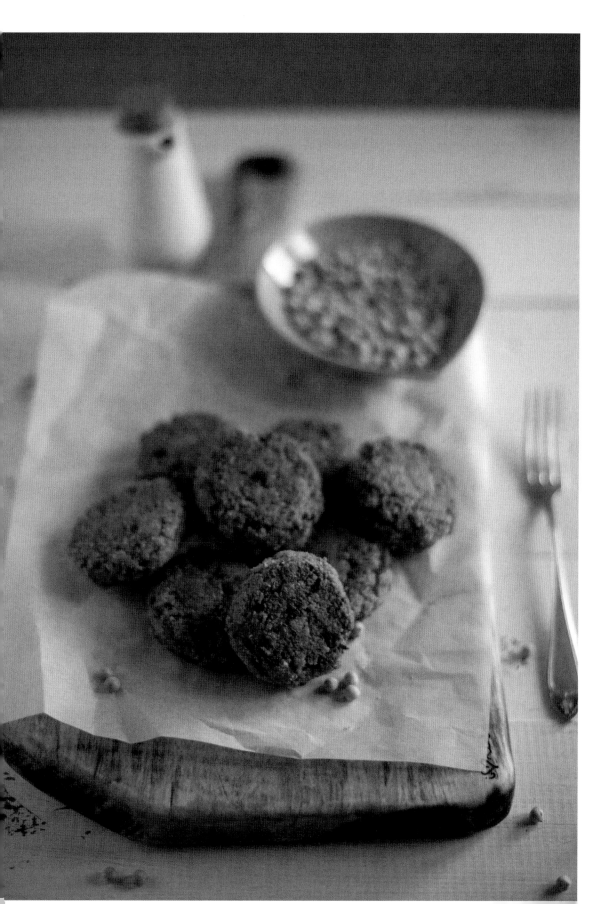

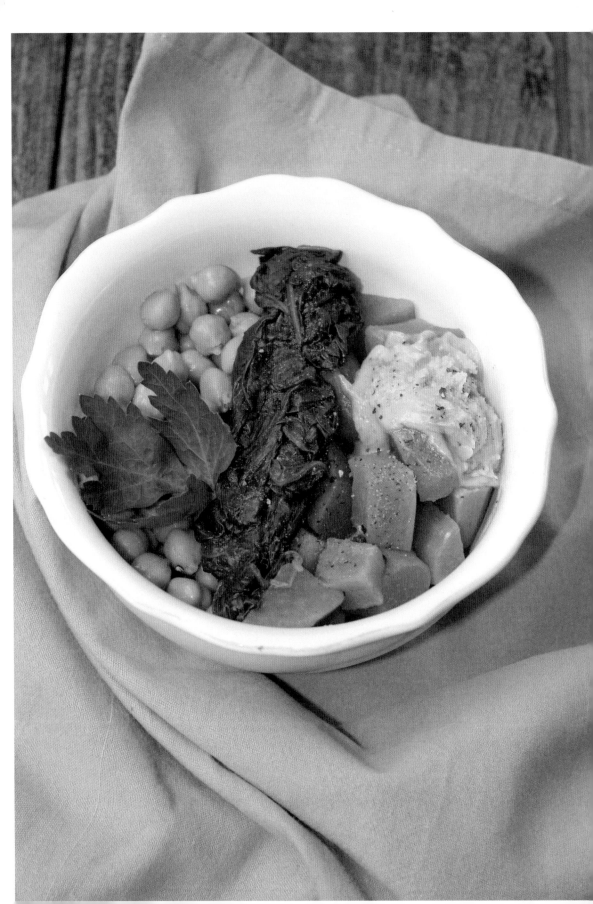

Super bowl

Serves 2

6 tbsp/80 g dried
chickpeas
2 medium/300 g sweet
potatoes
8 cups/300 g leaf
spinach
¾ inch/2 cm fresh
gingerroot
1 tbsp olive oil
½ tsp turmeric
2 cilantro stems
salt
freshly milled black
pepper
2 tbsp flax seed oil
2 tbsp peanut butter,
unsweetened

Soak the chickpeas overnight in plenty of water.
Drain in a sieve, rinse in fresh water, and place in
a saucepan with fresh water. Bring to a boil, then
cover and simmer over a low heat. Check to see if
the chickpeas are cooked after 45 to 60 minutes.
Drain, then cover and keep warm.

Peel, wash, and dice the sweet potatoes. Cook in a
saucepan for 7 to 12 minutes until firm to the bite,
then drain.

Clean and wash the spinach, then spin dry. Cook
in a steamer basket or in boiling water until the
leaves wilt, then keep warm. Peel, finely grate, or
chop the gingerroot.

Heat the olive oil in a saucepan or skillet. Brown
the sweet potatoes and gingerroot for a few
minutes, then season with the turmeric.

Wash the cilantro, then pat dry. Tear off and finely
chop the leaves. Divide the chickpeas, spinach,
and sweet potatoes between 2 bowls, season with
salt and pepper, then drizzle flax seed oil over the
top and serve garnished with cilantro leaves and
the peanut butter.

Lentils with oven-baked vegetables, chorizo, and apricots

Serves 4

3–4 small red onions
(or 8 red scallions if possible)
1 garlic bulb
1 hot, spicy chorizo
3 tbsp olive oil
sea salt
1 chile
1½ cups/350 ml vegetable stock
1 cup/200 g red lentils
juice of 2 limes
4 apricots
garam masala
pepper
bunch of parsley

Pre-heat the oven to 350 °F (180 °C). Peel and quarter the onions. Separate the garlic bulb into individual cloves but do not peel. Cut the chorizo into thin slices.

Spread the onions, garlic, and chorizo on a baking sheet lined with parchment paper. Drizzle with the oil, sprinkle with sea salt, and bake in the pre-heated oven for 20 minutes.

Wash the chile and slice into thin rings. Add the chile to the vegetable stock in a saucepan and bring to a boil, then add the lentils. Add half the lime juice, cover, and cook over a low heat.

Wash and pit the apricots, then cut each one into eight. Add to the vegetables in the oven for the last 5 minutes of cooking time.

Wash the parsley, shake dry and chop finely. Combine the lentils, oven-cooked vegetables, and chorizo, then season to taste with garam masala, pepper, and lime juice. Stir in the chopped parsley. Salted, natural yogurt makes a delicious accompaniment to this dish.

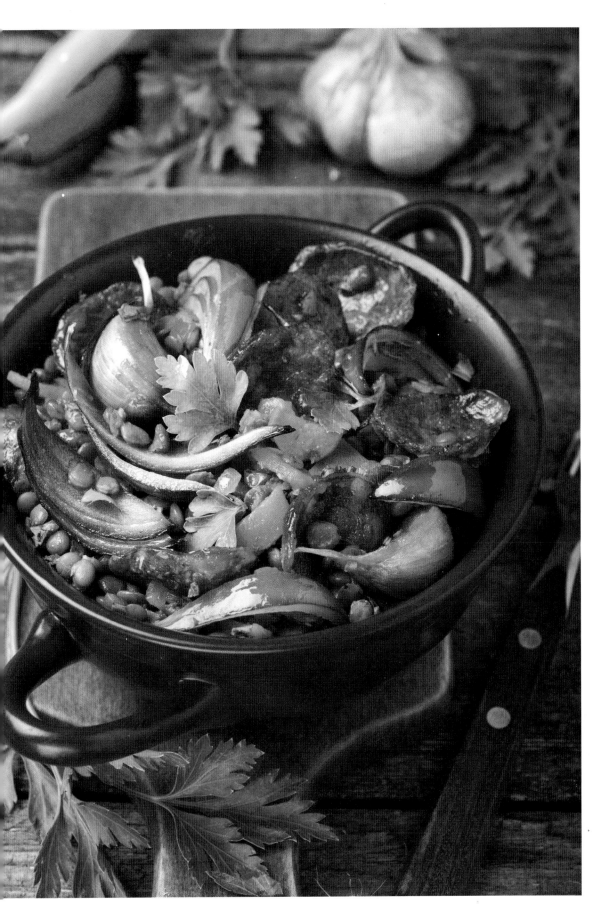

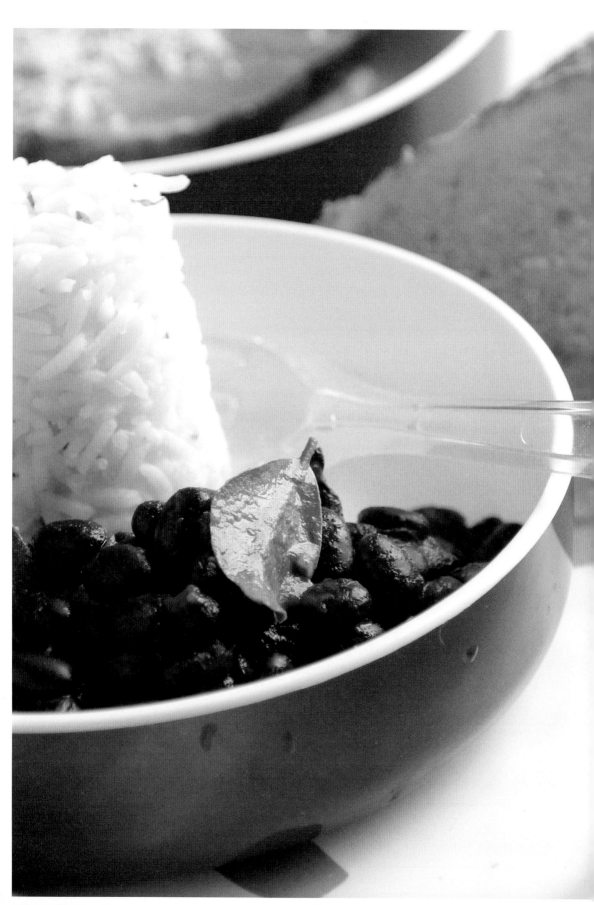

Brazilian feijoada

Serves 2

1 cup/200 g black, red,
or brown beans
2–3 garlic cloves
1 onion
1 chile
100 g "Kasseler" (pork
loin, salt-cured and
boned)
1 tbsp olive oil
2 cups/500 ml water
3 bay leaves
salt

Soak the beans for one day or overnight, then drain in a sieve and rinse in running water.

Peel and finely chop the garlic cloves, peel and finely dice the onion. Wash and clean the chile, then seed, if so desired, and slice into thin rings.

Cube the pork loin or slice into strips. Heat the olive oil in a saucepan, then brown the garlic, onion, chile, and pork loin over a medium heat for about 5 minutes, stirring frequently. Add the beans, water, and bay leaves and season to taste with salt.

Half cover the feijoada and simmer for at least one hour over a low heat. Meanwhile, add a little water, as required.

Tip

In Brazil, feijoada is usually served with an accompaniment of rice, but a chunk of white bread also goes well with this dish. I like this bean stew best when it includes cured pork loin and fresh horseradish.

Chili sin carne

Serves 4

3¼ cups/750 ml vegetable stock
4 oz/125 g soy mince (TVP)
about 3 medium/300 g waxy potatoes
1 onion
2 garlic cloves
1–2 chiles
2 tbsp olive oil
1 tbsp tomato paste
pinch of cinnamon
½ tsp cocoa powder, unsweetened
1 tbsp sweet paprika powder
1 tsp smoked paprika powder
sprig of fresh thyme
sprig of fresh marjoram
1 can kidney beans
1 red bell pepper
3 scallions
salt, pepper

Bring the vegetable stock to a boil and cook the soy mince for 5 minutes. Remove from the hob and leave to stand in the liquid until ready to use.

Peel and dice the potatoes and onion. Peel the garlic cloves, remove the green core, and roughly chop. Wash and chop the chile, and strip off the thyme and marjoram leaves.

Heat the oil in a large saucepan, then brown the onion and garlic. Add the diced potato and tomato paste and fry briefly.

Stir in the cinnamon, cocoa powder, both types of paprika powder, herbs, soy mince, and stock. Cover and simmer for about 10 minutes.

Next, add the kidney beans (along with their canning juice if desired) and simmer uncovered for 10 minutes.

Meanwhile, clean and dice the red bell pepper. Add to the chili mixture a short while before the chili is ready. Season with salt and pepper.

Clean the scallions, slice into rings, then sprinkle over the chili just before serving.

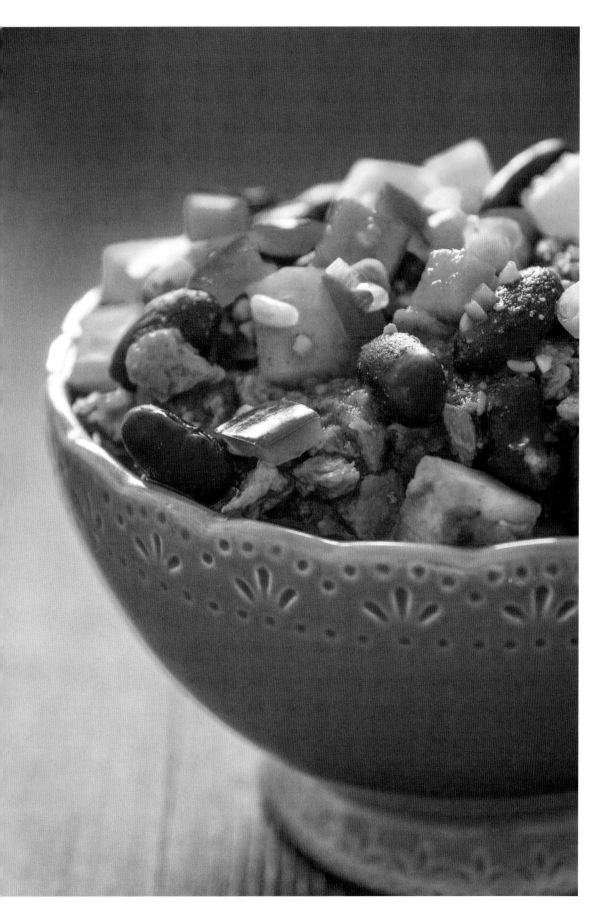

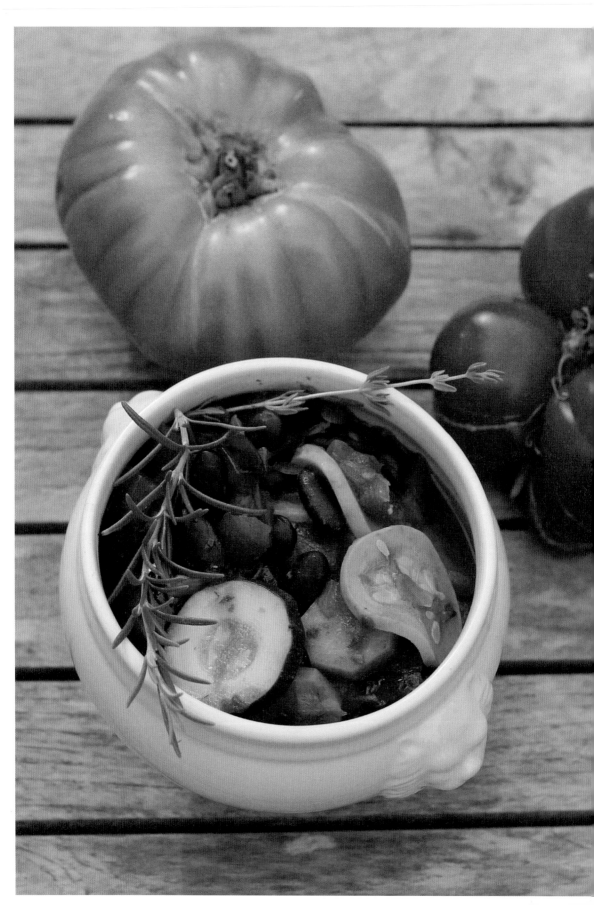

Ratatouille with kidney beans

Serves 2

1 cup/200 g dried
kidney beans
½ eggplant
1 zucchini
3 medium/400 g
tomatoes
1 bell pepper
1 carrot
1 onion
4 tbsp olive oil
1 cup/200 ml vegetable
stock
1 garlic clove
bunch of "herbes de
Provence"
1 cup/50 g dried
tomatoes
salt
freshly milled black
pepper

Soak the dried kidney beans for 12 hours in plenty of water. Drain the beans, then place in a saucepan of fresh water and bring to a boil. Simmer the beans for 45 minutes over a medium heat.

Meanwhile, clean and wash the eggplant, zucchini, fresh tomatoes, bell pepper, and carrot. Peel the carrot and seed the bell pepper. Cut the vegetables into bite-sized pieces. Peel and finely dice the onion.

Heat the olive oil in a saucepan, then sweat the onions until translucent. Add the vegetables and sweat for 2 to 3 minutes. Pour in the vegetable stock and simmer for another 15 minutes over a medium heat.

Peel and crush the garlic, wash the herbs and pat dry. Strip off and finely chop the leaves. Cut the dried tomatoes into thin strips. Lastly, add the kidney beans, dried tomatoes, garlic, and herbs, heat all the ingredients briefly, then season to taste with salt and pepper.

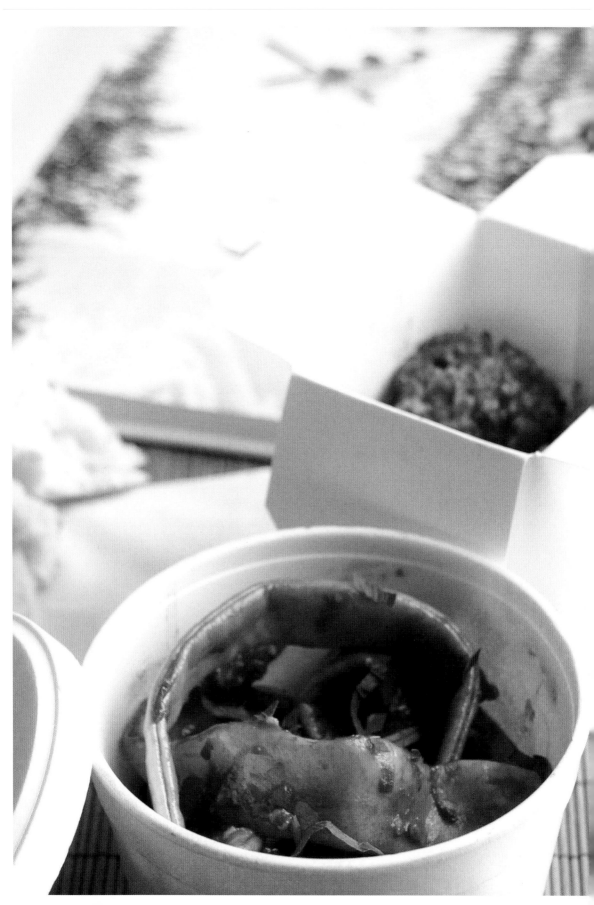

Green beans in tomato sauce with bulgur wheat

Serves 2

1 onion
3 garlic cloves
1 chile
1–2 tbsp olive oil
1¾ cups/400 g tomato purée
½ cup/100 ml water
1 tbsp raw cane sugar
salt
½ tsp cinnamon
2 cups/250 g green beans
½ cup/100 g bulgur wheat
2 tbsp marjoram, lovage, and peppermint
salt

Peel and dice the onion. Peel and finely chop the garlic cloves. Wash and clean the chile, then seed, if required, and slice into thin rings.

Heat the olive oil in a saucepan. Brown the onion, garlic, and chile, stirring occasionally. Add the tomato purée and water.

Season with sugar, salt, and cinnamon, then cover and simmer the tomato sauce for about 20 minutes over a gentle heat. Wash and clean the beans, top and tail, then cook in the sauce for about 20 minutes until tender.

Pour ½ cup/100 ml of boiling water over the bulgur wheat. Finely chop the marjoram, lovage, and mint, then stir into the sauce. Cover and cook for 5 to 10 minutes, then season with salt.

Lentil dal with peanuts

Serves 4

1 onion
2 garlic cloves
¾ inch/2 cm fresh
gingerroot
1 chile
1 sweet potato
1 carrot
3 tbsp oil
pinch of Madras curry
powder
pinch of turmeric
powder
pinch of cardamom
powder
1¼ cups/250 g red
lentils
½ cup/50 g raisins
½ tsp salt
juice of ½ lime
⅔ cup/100 g unsalted
shelled peanuts

Peel and finely chop the onion, garlic, and gingerroot. Cut the chile in half, remove the core and seeds, and slice into thin strips.

Peel the sweet potato and dice into roughly ⅓-inch/1-cm cubes. Peel the carrot, cut in half lengthwise, and slice into ¼-inch/0.5-cm chunks.

Heat the oil in a large saucepan and sweat the onion, gingerroot, garlic, and chile. Add the spices and red lentils, then continue to sweat all the ingredients for another 5 minutes, stirring constantly until the lentils are slightly translucent.

Add the sweet potato, carrot, and raisins, stirring constantly. Pour in about 3 cups/750 ml of warm water, then stir in the salt and lime juice.

Cover the saucepan with a lid and continue to simmer the dal for about 40 minutes. If all liquid gets absorbed before the lentils are cooked, add some warm water, a little at a time. The lentils should be soft but still firm to the bite.

Once the dal is ready, season to taste once more. Stir in the peanuts just before serving and serve with a green salad.

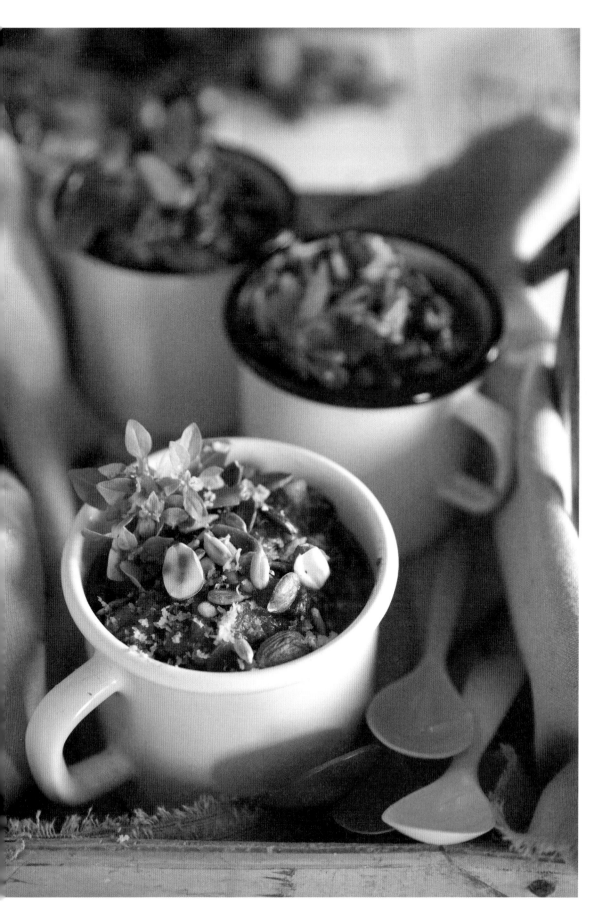

Asian vegetables in coconut sauce

Serves 4

½ cup/50 g green
beans
1 cup/100 g each
of broccoli and
cauliflower rosettes
1½ cups/100 g small
button mushrooms
5–6 oz/150 g turkey
breast fillets
¾ cup/100 g pineapple
6 scallions
1 garlic clove
1 red, sweet, pointed
pepper
1 tsp coconut oil
1 cup/100 g frozen
peas
1⅔ cups/400 ml
coconut milk
2 tbsp soy sauce
1 tbsp sesame seeds

Clean the green beans and cut into bite-sized
pieces. Blanch for about 5 minutes along with the
broccoli and cauliflower, then drain.

Clean and quarter the mushrooms. Rinse the
turkey fillets, pat dry, then cut into bite-sized
pieces. Dice the pineapple.

Wash and clean the scallions, then slice into rings.
Peel and crush the garlic. Wash, seed the sweet
red pepper, and slice into rings.

Heat the coconut oil in a skillet. Sauté the scallions
and garlic briefly, then add the meat and brown for
5 minutes.

Add the prepared vegetables, pineapple, peas, and
mushrooms, then brown for another 5 minutes,
stirring constantly.

Lastly, add the coconut milk and soy sauce, and
simmer for 10 minutes. Serve with rice.

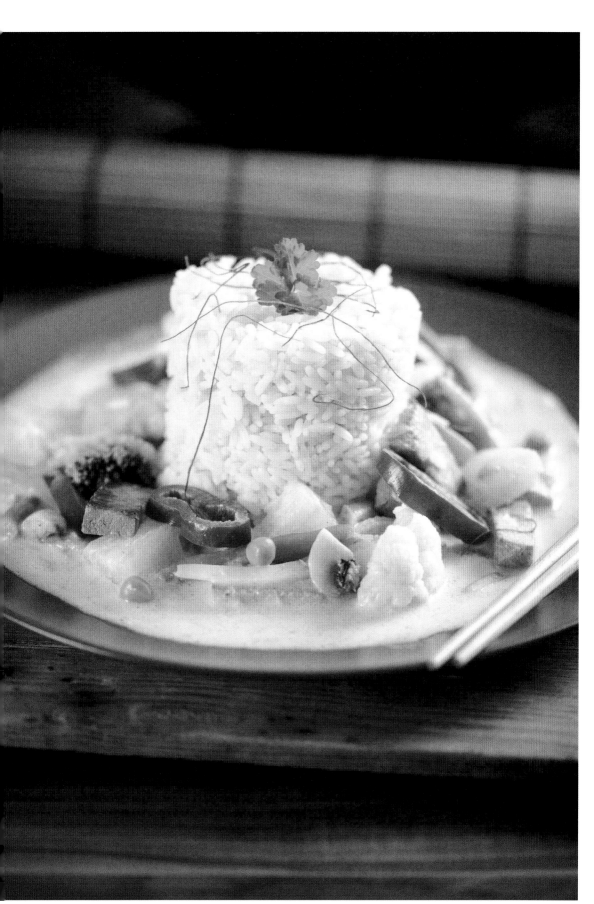

Bean stew with cilantro and peanuts

Serves 4

2½ cups/500 g mixed, dried beans
1 leek
¼ celery root (celeriac)
1 large carrot
3¼ cups/¾ l water
½ tsp salt
2¼ lb/1 kg potatoes
1 large onion
½ tsp turmeric
½ tsp ground coriander
salt, freshly milled black pepper
juice and grated zest of 1 lime
1 cinnamon stick
½ bunch cilantro
1 cup/150 g peanuts

Soak the dried beans overnight in cold water.

Wash and finely dice the leek, celery root, and carrot, then place in a large saucepan along with the water and salt. Simmer for about 1½ hours until the ingredients boil down into a hearty stock.

Meanwhile, drain the beans, rinse, put into a saucepan and cover with fresh water. Cook the beans for about 1 hour until just firm to the bite, then drain.

Peel and dice the potatoes and onion. Add to the stock along with the cooked beans, then season with turmeric, ground coriander, the lime zest and juice, and salt and pepper to taste. Add the cinnamon stick and cook the stew for a further 15 minutes.

Meanwhile, wash the cilantro, shake dry and finely chop. Toast the peanuts in a non-stick, fat-free skillet until they begin to release their aroma. Before serving, mix the peanuts and some of the cilantro into the stew. Serve sprinkled with the rest of the cilantro.

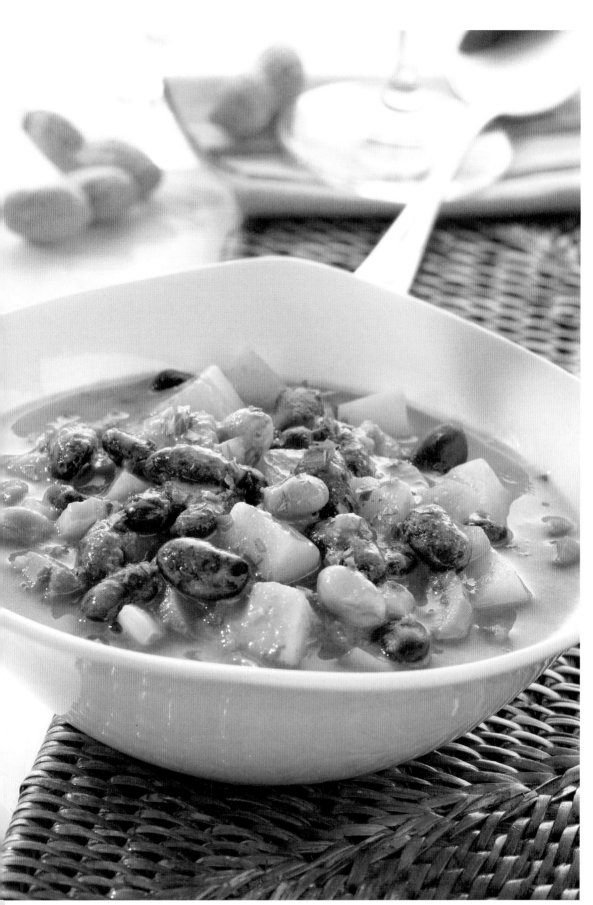

Wild rice with raisins, chickpeas, and cilantro

Serves 4

1 cup/200 g wild rice
1 tsp salt
1 large onion
½ inch/1 cm fresh gingerroot
1 can chickpeas
2 tbsp oil
1 tsp sugar
½ tsp salt
pinch of harissa
1 tsp red curry powder
pinch of cumin
pinch of turmeric
1 cup/100 g raisins
bunch of cilantro

Tip
This dish is perfect for using up rice cooked the previous day. Dried apricots or cranberries may be used as an alternative to raisins.

Bring the rice to a boil in double the quantity of water. Add the salt, cover and cook over a low heat for about 35–45 minutes. When cooked, the rice should be light and fluffy in the pan. Transfer the rice to a bowl and leave to cool.

Peel and finely chop the onion and gingerroot. Place the chickpeas in a sieve, rinse in cold water, then drain.

Heat the oil in a large skillet. Sear the onion and gingerroot quickly over a high heat. Add the sugar, then heat until slightly caramelized. Add the salt, harissa, curry powder, cumin, and turmeric, then brown all the ingredients, stirring constantly.

Add the chickpeas to the skillet, and mix well. Add the raisins and continue to stir. The spices and sugar make the rest of the ingredients susceptible to burning.

Add the wild rice. Stir all the ingredients well, then season with salt or add more hot spices, to taste. Finely chop the cilantro and sprinkle over the rice just before serving.

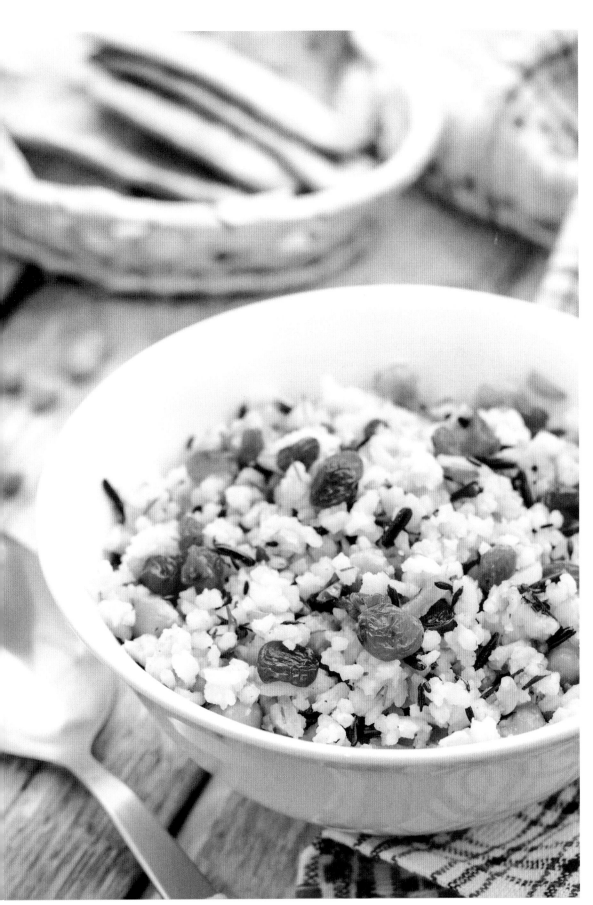

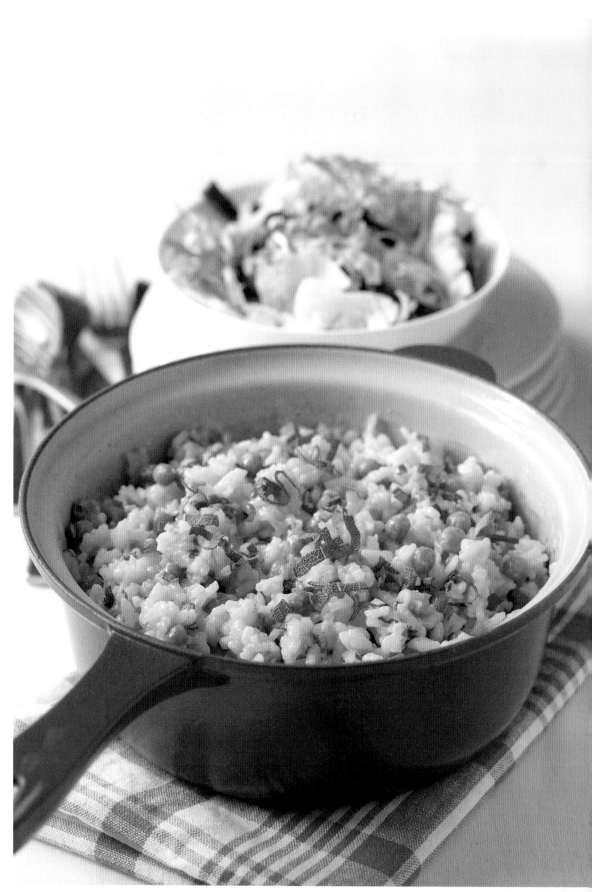

Pea risotto with mint

Serves 4

1 tbsp olive oil
2 onions
2 cups/400 g risotto
rice
1 cup/200 ml dry, white
wine
4 cups/1 liter vegetable
stock
2¼ cups/200 g sugar
snap peas
2 cups/250 g peas
4 oz/125 g piece of
Parmesan
bunch of basil
1 peppermint stem
5 tbsp/70 g butter
salt, freshly milled
black pepper
dash of lemon juice

Heat the oil in a saucepan. Peel, finely chop the onions, and sweat in the oil until translucent, then add the rice. Cook for a few minutes, then pour in the wine. Top up with vegetable stock and simmer for about 15 minutes, stirring regularly to prevent the rice sticking.

Remove any stringy strands from the sugar snap peas and cut into thin strips. Add to the risotto along with the peas 6 minutes before the rice is ready. The rice should be soft but still firm to the bite. Finely chop the herbs, grate the Parmesan, and blend into the risotto along with the butter. Season to taste with salt, pepper, and some lemon juice.

Squash stuffed with borage

Serves 4

12 small round squash
(about 2–2½ in/5–7 cm)
or Patisson squash
1 tbsp oil
bunch of parsley
chives
small bunch/50 g
borage
1 cup/200 g dried
chickpeas or chickpea
purée
salt, freshly milled
black pepper
borage flowers, to
garnish
almond butter or
cashew paste, to taste

Soak the dried chickpeas, ideally overnight. Next day, drain, rinse, and boil the chickpeas in fresh, salted water, then purée.

Wash and dry the squash, then scoop out the flesh.

Wash, dry, and chop the herbs. Mix the herbs and chickpea purée together and season to taste with salt and pepper.

Pre-heat the oven to 340 °F (170 °C). Spoon the mixture into the squash shells, then arrange in a baking dish, replace the lids to begin with, then bake in the pre-heated oven for 30 minutes.

Spread the almond butter over the squash and bake in the pre-heated oven with the lids removed for a further 10 minutes to brown the filling.

These miniature squashes can also be topped with cheese, as shown here in the photograph.

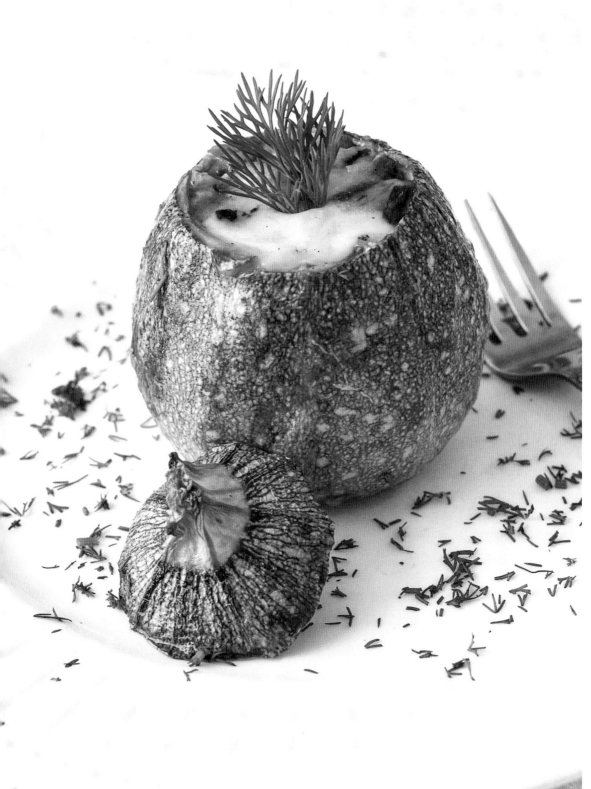

Index

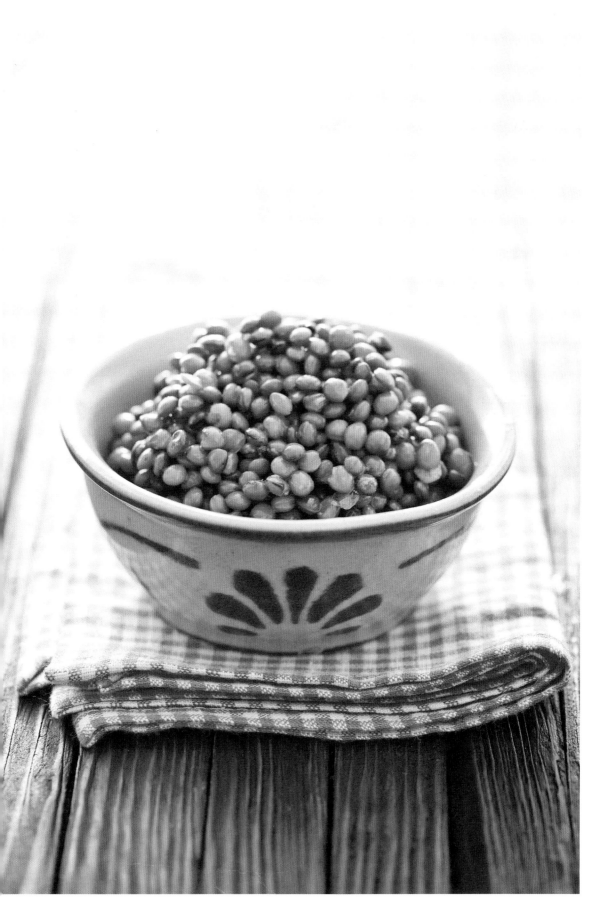

Abbreviations and Quantities

1 oz = 1 ounce = 28 grams
1 lb = 1 pound = 16 ounces
1 cup = approx. 5–8 ounces* (see below)
1 cup = 8 fluid ounces = 250 milliliters (liquids)
2 cups = 1 pint (liquids) = 500 milliliters (liquids)
8 pints = 4 quarts = 1 gallon (liquids)
1 g = 1 gram = 1/1000 kilogram = 5 ml (liquids)
1 kg = 1 kilogram = 1000 grams = 2¼ lb
1 l = 1 liter = 1000 milliliters (ml) = 1 quart
125 milliliters (ml) = approx. 8 tablespoons = ½ cup
1 tbsp = 1 level tablespoon = 15–20 g* (depending on density) = 15 milliliters (liquids)
1 tsp = 1 level teaspoon = 3–5 g * (depending on density) = 5 ml (liquids)
*The weight of dry ingredients varies significantly depending on the density factor, e.g. 1 cup of flour weighs less than 1 cup of butter. Quantities in ingredients have been rounded up or down for convenience, where appropriate. Metric conversions may therefore not correspond exactly. It is important to use either American or metric measurements within a recipe.

Picture credits

Fotolia: Front Cover, back cover, PP. 6, 11, 13, 14, 17, 19, 20, 23, 24, 27, 28, 31, 51, 54, 58, 83, 84, 89, 91, 93, 95, 96, 99, 105, 109, 113, 117, 121, 125, 131, 133, 137, 141, 143
Hannah Frey: PP. 37, 45, 49, 53, 60, 86, 106, 114, 118, 126
Sarah Golbaz: PP. 77
Mauritius Images: PP. 32
Martina Schurich: PP. 64, 67, 70, 73, 81, 103, 122, 128
Stockfood: PP. 39, 40, 42, 46, 57, 63, 68, 74, 78, 100, 110, 135, 138
Maiga Werner: PP. 34

Disclaimer

© for the original edition: h.f.ullmann publishing GmbH
Original title: *Hülsenfrüchte! Power-Rezepte mit Bohnen, Erbsen, Linsen & Co.*

Original ISBN: 978-3-8480-1034-9

Concept, Editing, Layout, Cover design: Christine Paxmann text • konzept • grafik, München
Text: Hannah Frey (PP. 36, 44, 48, 52, 61, 87, 107, 115, 119, 127), Sarah Golbaz (PP. 41, 76), Christian Havenith (PP. 43, 47, 134, 139), Marion Koschkar (PP. 7–13, 21, 25, 26, 82, 104, 112, 124, 132), Christine Paxmann (PP. 50, 55, 56, 69, 90, 94, 98, 108, 120, 130, 136), Antje Radcke (PP. 18, 22, 29, 30, 111), Martina Schurich (PP. 38, 62–66, 71–75, 79–80, 88, 92, 101, 102, 123, 129), Maiga Werner (PP. 35, 116, 140) and Ute-Marion Wilkesmann (P. 16)
Project management for h.f.ullmann: Martin Dort, Lars Pietzschmann

© for this English edition: h.f.ullmann publishing GmbH

Translation from German: Susan Ghanouni in association with First Edition Translations Ltd, Cambridge, UK
Editing: Lin Thomas in association with First Edition Translations Ltd, Cambridge, UK
Typesetting: The Write Idea Ltd in association with First Edition Translations Ltd, Cambridge, UK

Printed in Germany, 2016

Overall responsibility for production: h.f.ullmann publishing, Potsdam, Germany

ISBN 978-3-8480-1035-6

10 9 8 7 6 5 4 3 2 1
X IX VIII VII VI V IV III II I

www.ullmannmedien.com
info@ullmannmedien.com
facebook.com/ullmannmedien
twitter.com/ullmann_int

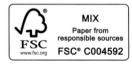

FSC
www.fsc.org

MIX
Paper from
responsible sources
FSC® C004592